DIY Home Face Mask And Hand Sanitizer

Unfu*k Germs and Bacteria and Prevent Yourself and Your Family from Common Flu and other Viral Diseases.

By Johnson Pfizer

Table of Contents

DO IT YOURSELF HOMEMADE FACE MASK

HOMEMADE HAND SANITIZER

DO IT YOURSELF HOMEMADE FACE MASK

By Johnson Pfizer

Table of Contents

Introduction

Wearing a face mask in public areas may impede the spread of an infectious disease by preventing both the inhalation of infectious droplets and their subsequent exhalation

and dissemination. In the event of a pandemic involving an airborne-transmissible agent, the general public will have limited access to the type of high- level respiratory protection worn by health care workers, such as N95 respirators. Images of members of the public wearing surgical masks were often used to illustrate the 2009 H1N1 flu pandemic. However, the evidence of proportionate benefit from widespread use of face masks is unclear.

A recent prospective cluster-randomized trial comparing surgical masks and non-fit-tested P2 masks (filters at least 94% of airborne particles) with no mask use in the prevention of influenza-like illness. The findings of the study found that adherence to mask use significantly reduced (95%) the risk for infection associated with influenza-like illness which include the just discovered Covid-19, but that less than 50% of participants wore masks most of the time.

Facemasks may prevent contamination of the work space during the outbreak of influenza or other droplet-spread communicable disease by reducing aerosol transmission. They may also be used to reduce the risk of body fluids, including blood, secretions, and excretions, from reaching the wearer's mouth and nose.

To date, studies on the efficacy and reliability of face masks have concentrated on their use by health care workers.

Although health care workers are likely to be one of the highest risk groups in terms of exposure,they are also more likely to be trained in the use of masks and fit tested than the general public. Should the supply of standard commercial face masks not meet demand, it would be useful to know whether improvised masks could provide any protection to others from those who are infected and that include homemade face mask.

In this ebook we will discuss more on the uses of face mask and every other things you must know about the benefit of homemade face mask as well as how to make a good and affordable face mask for you and your family.

Wearing a medical mask is one of the prevention measures to limit spread of certain respiratory diseases, including 2019-nCoV, in affected areas. However, the use of a mask alone is insufficient to provide the adequate level of protection and other equally relevant measures should be adopted.If masks are to be used, this measure must be combined with hand hygiene and other IPC measures to prevent the human-to-human transmission of 2019-nCov.WHO has developed guidance for home care band health care settings con infection prevention and control(IPC) strategies for use when infection with 2019-nCoV is suspected. Wearing medical masks when not indicated may cause unnecessary cost, procurement burden and create a false sense of security that can lead to neglecting other essential measures such as hand hygiene practices.Furthermore, using a mask incorrectly may hamper its effectiveness to reduce the risk of transmission.

Chapter 1

What is Face mask?

A face mask is a device that you wear over your face, for example to prevent yourself from breathing bad air or from spreading germs, or to protect your face when you are in a dangerous situation.

Face masks are one tool utilized for preventing the spread of disease. They may also be called dental, isolation, laser, medical, procedure, or surgical masks. Face masks are loose-fitting masks that cover the nose and mouth, and have ear loops or ties or bands at the back of the head. There are many different brands and they come in different colors. It is important to use a face mask approved by the FDA.

Wearing a face mask is certainly not an iron-clad guarantee that you won't get sick – viruses can also transmit through the eyes and tiny viral particles, known as aerosols, can penetrate masks. However, masks are effective at capturing droplets, which is a main transmission route of coronavirus, and some studies have estimated a roughly fivefold protection versus no barrier alone (although others have found lower levels of effectiveness).

If you are likely to be in close contact with someone infected, a mask cuts the chance of the disease being passed on. If you're showing symptoms of coronavirus, or have been diagnosed, wearing a mask can also protect others. So masks are crucial for health and social care workers looking after patients and are also recommended for family members who need to care for someone who is ill – ideally both the patient and carer should have a mask.

However, masks will probably make little difference if you're just walking around town or taking a bus so there is no need to bulk-buy a huge supply.

Uses of Face Mask

Face mask provides a physical barrier to fluids and large particle droplets. Surgical mask is a type of face mask commonly used. When used properly, surgical masks can prevent infections transmitted by respiratory droplets.

Since the beginning of the global coronavirus pandemic, Americans have been told by the Centers for Disease Control and Prevention not to wear masks unless they are sick, caring for a sick person who is unable to wear one or working in health care.

Numerous reasons have been given: that they don't offer significant protection from germs, that the most effective models need special fitting in order to work, that regular people don't typically wear them correctly, that they'll give people a false sense of security and cause them to be lax about hand-washing and social distancing.

And most of all: that there aren't enough masks and respirators for the health-care workers who desperately need them so leave the masks to them.

Now there are big changes to that policy.

The Trump administration announced Friday that the CDC is now recommending people consider wearing cloth face coverings in public settings where other social distancing measures are difficult to maintain. Mayors in New York City and Los Angeles have already offered similar advice to citizens. In this ebook we are still going to discuss about cloth face mask and its efficiency.

There's one big reason for the change: There is increasing evidence that virus and other influenza can be spread by presymptomatic and asymptomatic carriers.

These new policies come with the vital plea that people don't use the medical-grade masks that are in short supply in hospitals. That means one thing: The era of the homemade masks and face coverings is upon us.

With this new attitude come many questions — which we'll attempt to answer here.

When to Wear face mask?

The purpose of all of us wearing face coverings or surgical masks anywhere people congregate is first and foremost to protect others if we sneeze or cough. These coverings will stop much of the large droplets that could otherwise reach people as far away as 18 feet away. Just-published research indicates that surgical masks can also decrease the amount of aerosolized virus the people produce by breathing and talking.

A big question is: Can these DIY or surgical masks also protect the wearer? The same research study shows these masks impede aerosolized virus being expelled out by the user so presumably they can decrease breathing in the virus, influenza or any other causative agent as well. But they aren't foolproof. These coverings don't fit the face tightly, so aerosolized virus and larger droplets can be sucked in through the gaps between the face and the mask when we take a breath.

Additionally, some of the viral particles are so small that they can be inhaled through the cloth or paper that's used to make these masks. People should not be lulled into a false sense of security in thinking that these types of masks will protect them from airborne, aerosolized virus especially in poorly ventilated spaces frequented by others. The best thing to do is to either avoid such spaces or be in them for as short a period of time as possible.

Wearing face coverings is recommended and requested for when you are indoors, including mass transit and ride-shares, with other people.

Anywhere you go, maintain physical distancing of at least 6 feet with no bodily contact. If someone nearby sneezes or coughs and they aren't wearing a mask, get at least 20 feet away, quickly. When you do go out on an errand, wear a face covering and get your business done as fast as you can.

You don't need an N95 mask if you wear a face covering when you go out in a public indoor place or ride mass transit and practice good physical distancing. Health care workers have to care for their patients within very close distances for prolonged periods of time. If they don't have an N95 mask, the risk goes way up for them.

Types of Face Mask

N95 respirators and surgical masks (face masks) are examples of personal protective equipment that are used to protect the wearer from airborne particles and from liquid contaminating the face. Centers for Disease Control and Prevention (CDC) National Institute for Occupational Safety and Health (NIOSH) and Occupational Safety and Health Administration (OSHA) also regulate N95 respirators.

It is important to recognize that the optimal way to prevent airborne transmission is to use a combination of interventions from across the hierarchy of controls,

Surgical Masks (Face Masks)

A surgical mask is a disposable medical device that can be bought in pharmacy and that protects against infectious agents transmitted by "droplets." These droplets can be droplets of saliva or secretions from the upper respiratory tract when the wearer exhales.

If worn by the caregiver, the surgical mask protects the patient and his or her environment (air, surfaces, equipment, surgical site). If worn by a contagious patient, it prevents the patient from contaminating his or her surroundings and environment. These masks should not be worn for more than 3 to 8 hours.

A surgical mask can also protect the wearer from the risk of splashes of biological fluids. In this case, the surgical mask must have a waterproof layer. It can also be equipped with a visor to protect the eyes.

But a surgical mask does not protect against "airborne" infectious agents so it will not prevent the wearer from being potentially contaminated by a virus such as the coronavirus.

A surgical mask is a loose-fitting, disposable device that creates a physical barrier between the mouth and nose of the wearer and potential contaminants in the immediate environment. Surgical masks are regulated under 21 CFR 878.4040. Surgical masks are not to be shared and may be labeled as surgical, isolation, dental, or medical procedure face masks. They may come with or without a face shield. These are often referred to as face masks, although not all face masks are regulated as surgical masks.

Surgical masks are made in different thicknesses and with different ability to protect you from contact with liquids. These properties may also affect how easily you can breathe through the face mask and how well the surgical mask protects you.

If worn properly, a surgical mask is meant to help block large-particle droplets, splashes, sprays, or splatter that may contain germs (viruses and bacteria), keeping it from reaching your mouth and nose. Surgical masks may also help reduce exposure of your saliva and respiratory secretions to others.

While a surgical mask may be effective in blocking splashes and large-particle droplets, a face mask, by design, does not filter or block very small particles in the air that may be transmitted by coughs, sneezes, or certain medical procedures. Surgical masks also do not provide complete protection from germs and other contaminants because of the loose fit between the surface of the face mask and your face.

Surgical masks are not intended to be used more than once. If your mask is damaged or soiled, or if breathing through the mask becomes difficult, you should remove the face mask, discard it safely, and replace it with a new one. To safely discard your mask, place it in a plastic bag and put it in the trash. Wash your hands after handling the used mask.

N95 Respirators

An N95 respirator is a respiratory protective device designed to achieve a very close facial fit and very efficient filtration of airborne particles.

The 'N95' designation means that when subjected to careful testing, the respirator blocks at least 95 percent of very small (0.3 micron) test particles. If properly fitted, the filtration capabilities of N95 respirators exceed those of face masks. However, even a properly fitted N95 respirator does not completely eliminate the risk of illness or death.

The right way to wear and remove face mask?

People should wear a surgical mask when they have respiratory infection; when taking care of patient with respiratory infection; or when visiting clinics or hospitals during pandemic or peak season for influenza in order to reduce the spread of infection.

Points to note on wearing a Face mask:

(a)Choose the appropriate mask size. Child size is available for selection as indicated.

(b)Perform hand hygiene before putting on a surgical mask.

(c)The surgical mask should fit snugly over the face:

(i)Most surgical masks adopt a three-layer design (Annex I) which includes an outer fluid-repelling layer, a middle layer serves as a barrier to germs, and an inner moisture-absorbing layer. Mask without the above functions is not recommended as it cannot provide adequate protection against infectious diseases transmitted by respiratory droplets. Wearer should follow the manufacturers' recommendations when using surgical mask, including proper storage and procedures of putting on surgical mask (e.g. determine which side of the mask is facing outwards). In general,the coloured side/the side with folds facing downwards of the surgical mask should face outwards with the metallic strip uppermost.

(ii)For tie-on surgical mask, secure upper ties at the crown of head. Then secure lower ties at the nape. For ear-loops type, position the elastic bands around both ears.

(iii)Extend the surgical mask to fully cover mouth, nose and chin(Image 3).

(iv)Mould the metallic strip over nose bridge and the surgical mask should fit snugly over the face(Image 4).

(d)Avoid touching the surgical mask after wearing. Otherwise, should perform hand hygiene before and after touching the mask.

(e)When taking off tie-on surgical mask, unfasten the ties at the nape first; then unfasten the ties at the crown of head(image 5). For ear-loops type, hold both the ear loops and take-off gently from face.

Avoid touching the outside of surgical mask during taking-off as it may be covered with germs.

(f)After taking off the surgical mask, discard in a lidded rubbish bin and perform hand hygiene immediately.

(g)Change surgical mask timely. In general, surgical mask should not be reused.Replace the mask immediately if it is damaged or soiled.

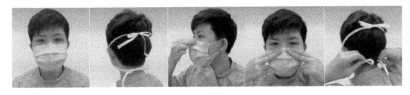

Image 1   Image 2   Image 3   Image 4   Image 5

Before putting on a mask, clean hands with alcohol-based hand rub or soap and water.

Cover mouth and nose with mask and make sure there are no gaps between your face and the mask.

Avoid touching the mask while using it; if you do, clean your hands with alcohol-based hand rub or soap and water.

Replace the mask with a new one as soon as it is damp and do not re-use single-use masks.

To remove the mask: remove it from behind (do not touch the front of mask); discard immediately in a closed bin; clean hands with alcohol-based hand rub or soap and water.

Additional Recommendations on Use of Surgical Mask during Influenza Pandemic in the Community Setting

During Influenza Pandemic, apart from using surgical mask properly, we should adopt the following preventive measures vigilantly to minimize the risk of getting infection:

(a)Perform hand hygiene frequently and properly.

(b)Perform hand hygiene before touching eyes, nose and mouth.

(c)Maintain respiratory etiquette/cough manners(Picture below).

(d)Stay at home if got sick and minimize contact with others.

(e)Stay away from possible sources of infection:(i)Minimize unnecessary social contacts and avoid visiting crowded places. If this is necessary, minimize the length of stay whenever possible. Moreover, person at a high risk of having infection-related complications, e.g. pregnant woman or persons with chronic illnesses are advised to wear surgical mask.

(ii)Avoid close contact with the infected persons.

How to put on other type of face mask

Clean your hands with soap and water or hand sanitizer before touching the mask.

Remove a mask from the box and make sure there are no obvious tears or holes in either side of the mask.

Determine which side of the mask is the top. The side of the mask that has a stiff bendable edge is the top and is meant to mold to the shape of your nose.

Determine which side of the mask is the front. The colored side of the mask is usually the front and should face away from you, while the white side touches your face.

Follow the instructions below for the type of mask you are using.

Face Mask with Ear loops: Hold the mask by the ear loops. Place a loop around each ear.

Face Mask with Ties: Bring the mask to your nose level and place the ties over the crown of your head and secure with a bow.

Face Mask with Bands: Hold the mask in your hand with the nosepiece or top of the mask at fingertips, allowing the headbands to hang freely below hands. Bring the mask to your nose level and pull the top strap over your head so that it rests over the crown of your head. Pull the bottom strap over your head so that it rests at the nape of your neck.

Mold or pinch the stiff edge to the shape of your nose.

If using a face mask with ties: Then take the bottom ties, one in each hand, and secure with a bow at the nape of your neck.

Pull the bottom of the mask over your mouth and chin.

How to remove other face mask

Clean your hands with soap and water or hand sanitizer before touching the mask. Avoid touching the front of the mask. The front of the mask is contaminated. Only touch the ear loops/ties/band.Follow the instructions below for the type of mask you are using.

Face Mask with Ear loops: Hold both of the ear loops and gently lift and remove the mask.

Face Mask with Ties: Untie the bottom bow first then untie the top bow and pull the mask away from you as the ties are loosened.

Face Mask with Bands: Lift the bottom strap over your head first then pull the top strap over your head.

Throw the mask in the trash. Clean your hands with soap and water or hand sanitizer.

Chapter 2

Masks management

If medical masks are worn, appropriate use and disposal is essential to ensure they are effective and to avoid any increase in risk of transmission associated with the incorrect use and disposal of masks. The following information on correct use of medical masks derives from the practices in health-care setting.

1. place mask carefully to cover mouth and nose and tie securely to minimise any gaps between the face and the mask;- while in use, avoid touching the mask; -remove the mask by using appropriate technique (i.e. do not touch the front but remove the lace from behind); -after removal or whenever you in advertently touch a used mask, clean hands by using an alcohol-based hand rubor soap and water if visibly soiled- replace masks with a new clean, dry mask as soon as they become damp/humid;-do not re-use single-use masks;-discard single-use masks after each use and dispose of them immediately upon removal.Cloth(e.g. cotton or gauze) masks are not recommended under any circumstance.

Comparing Surgical Masks and Surgical N95 Respirators

The FDA regulates surgical masks and surgical N95 respirators differently based on their intended use.

A surgical mask is a loose-fitting, disposable device that creates a physical barrier between the mouth and nose of the wearer and potential contaminants in the immediate environment. These are often referred to as face masks, although not all face masks are regulated as surgical masks. Note that the edges of the mask are not designed to form a seal around the nose and mouth.

An N95 respirator is a respiratory protective device designed to achieve a very close facial fit and very efficient filtration of airborne particles. Note that the edges of the respirator are designed to form a seal around the nose and mouth. Surgical N95 Respirators are commonly used in healthcare settings and are a subset of N95 Filtering Facepiece Respirators (FFRs), often referred to as N95s.

The similarities among surgical masks and surgical N95s are:

They are tested for fluid resistance, filtration efficiency (particulate filtration efficiency and bacterial filtration efficiency), flammability and biocompatibility.

They should not be shared or reused.

General N95 Respirator Precautions

People with chronic respiratory, cardiac, or other medical conditions that make breathing difficult should check with their health care provider before using an N95 respirator because the N95 respirator can make it more difficult for the wearer to breathe. Some models have exhalation valves that can make breathing out easier and help reduce heat build-up. Note that N95 respirators with exhalation valves should not be used when sterile conditions are needed.

All FDA-cleared N95 respirators are labeled as "single-use," disposable devices. If your respirator is damaged or soiled, or if breathing becomes difficult, you should remove the respirator, discard it properly, and replace it with a new one. To safely discard your N95 respirator, place it in a plastic bag and put it in the trash. Wash your hands after handling the used respirator.

N95 respirators are not designed for children or people with facial hair. Because a proper fit cannot be achieved on children and people with facial hair, the N95 respirator may not provide full protection.

N95 Respirators in Industrial and Health Care Settings

Most N95 respirators are manufactured for use in construction and other industrial type jobs that expose workers to dust and small particles. They are regulated by the National Personal Protective Technology Laboratory (NPPTL) in the National Institute for Occupational Safety and Health (NIOSH), which is part of the Centers for Disease Control and Prevention (CDC)

However, some N95 respirators are intended for use in a health care setting. Specifically, single-use, disposable respiratory protective devices used and worn by health care personnel during procedures to protect both the patient and health care personnel from the transfer of microorganisms, body fluids, and particulate material. These surgical N95 respirators are class II devices regulated by the FDA, under 21 CFR 878.4040, and CDC NIOSH under 42 CFR Part 84.

N95s respirators regulated under product code MSH are class II medical devices exempt from 510(k) premarket notification, unless:

The respirator is intended to prevent specific diseases or infections, or

The respirator is labeled or otherwise represented as filtering surgical smoke or plumes, filtering specific amounts of viruses or bacteria, reducing the amount of and/or killing viruses, bacteria, or fungi, or affecting allergenicity, or

The respirator contains coating technologies unrelated to filtration (e.g., to reduce and or kill microorganisms).

Dental professionals should wear appropriate personal protective equipment—including masks, which adhere to Standard Precautions for protection of the mouth and nose—when splashes or sprays of blood and body fluids are likely.

Can face coverings prevent the spread of the virus?

The primary benefit of covering your nose and mouth is that you protect others. While there is still much to be learned about the novel coronavirus, it appears that many people who are infected are shedding the virus – through coughs, sneezes and other respiratory droplets – for 48 hours before they start feeling sick. And others who have the virus – up to 25%, according to Centers for Disease Control and Prevention Director Dr. Robert Redfield — may never feel symptoms but may still play a role in transmitting it.

That's why wearing a mask even if you don't feel sick can be a good idea.

If you cough or sneeze, the mask can catch those respiratory droplets so they don't land on other people or surfaces. "So it's not going to protect you, but it is going to protect your neighbor," says Dr. Daniel Griffin at Columbia University, an expert on infectious diseases. "If your neighbor is wearing a mask and the same thing happens, they're going to protect you. So masks worn properly have the potential to benefit people."

The best masks are N95 respirators, but the general public is urged not to use them because they are fiercely needed by health care workers right now. If you have those, consider donating them immediately to a local hospital or find a drop-off here. Same goes for surgical masks — those thin blue models-- which offer less protection but are helpful and are also in short supply.

If I'm wearing a mask and someone sneezes on me, would the mask offer some protection?

Yes. But only if you use the mask properly and don't touch it with your hands afterward.

Those droplets from a cough or sneeze would hit your mask instead of your mouth and nose — good news. But the next step is to take the mask off by the ear bands and either wash or discard it — without touching the front of it.

"That's what I see all the time," says Griffin. "That's why in the studies, masks fail — people don't use them [correctly]. They touch the front of it. They adjust it. They push it down somehow to get their nose stuck out."

If you touch the front of the mask, whatever that person coughed or sneezed on it is now on your hands.

As this video from the World Health Organization shows, you should take off your mask by removing the elastics or straps from behind your ears. Don't touch the front, and keep the mask away from your face.

One other thing: Ideally you would have eye protection, too, to keep that stranger's sneeze from getting in. Glasses and sunglasses aren't perfect but can help.

Chapter 3

What about homemade masks?

As NPR has previously reported, some research has shown that cotton T-shirt material and tea towels might help block respiratory droplets emitting from sick people — though it's not clear how much protection they provide.

Another study, of health care workers in Vietnam, found that use of cloth masks resulted in greater infection than either those wearing surgical masks or a control group, some of whom also wore surgical masks.

We don't yet know exactly how effective homemade masks are, but Griffin thinks they're a good idea — he has even taken to wearing one over his N95 respirator.

How often do I need to wash it?

Griffin says to think of a mask as like underwear: It needs to be washed after each use.

"You don't take this dirty mask off, put it in your purse and then stick it back on your face," he says. "It's something that once you put on, is potentially either touching your coughs, sneezes or the spray of your speech, or protecting you from the coughs, spray, speech of other people. And now it's dirty. It needs to basically be either discarded or washed."

So if you're wearing a cloth mask, put it into the laundry basket immediately. If it's disposable, throw it away.

It's a big no-no to pull the mask down to eat a snack, then pull it back up: You've just gotten whatever dirty stuff is on the mask on your hands and into your mouth.

Is there one best mask design?

There is little data so far on cloth or homemade masks in general — let alone data that dictates how many pleats to put on your home-sewn version.

Griffin says the best material to use is a tight-weave cotton. "Don't use a synthetic or a polyester because they've looked at the virus's ability to survive on surfaces, and spandex is the worst," he says.

Johns Hopkins Medicine has one design you might try. Kaiser Permanente has another design, as well as a video showing how to make a mask using a sewing machine. Both recommend 100% woven cotton fabric. Kaiser recommends washing and drying the fabric two or three times before cutting it, so it doesn't shrink later.

You can make a mask out of a T-shirt, no sewing machine required. You could also try making one out of (unused) shop towels. But no matter what you make it out of, try to make it fit closely to your face and don't touch the front of it once you've started wearing it.

If you use cloth masks, make a number of them so you can wear a fresh one each time you go out.

Would a scarf work?

Probably not as well as a mask that fits closely to your face.

"You can imagine if you put a loosely knit scarf with lots of holes in it ... that would not be very effective," says Dr. Michael Klompas, an infectious disease physician at Brigham and Women's Hospital.

The goal is to create a barrier that catches droplets and keeps others from coming in, so you want coverage that is tightly woven and close-fitting.

Do masks confer any other benefits?

Masks can also function as an important visual cue, says Joseph Allen, an assistant professor of exposure and assessment science at Harvard University T.H. Chan School of Public Health.

They're a "reminder that we need to be taking these precautions and serve as a reminder to people to keep that 6-foot buffer," he says. "It should be seen as a badge of honor. If I'm wearing a mask out in public, it means I'm concerned about you, I'm concerned about my neighbors, I'm concerned about strangers on the chance that I'm infectious. I want to do my part in limiting how I might impact you."

Klompas agrees — and says that it can also give the wearer a welcome sense of security.

"It feels like you're behind a shield," he says, "and I think that in itself can be reassuring."

And for the others around you, it's a warning. "It says: Watch out. There's a public health crisis right now, there's a virus going around, we need to be on top guard," says Klompas. "I think it can actually be a reinforcer, a reminder of the state of crisis that we face in society."

But he says that masks are not a replacement for all the other steps we need to take right now to protect ourselves from the coronavirus — especially social distancing and good hand hygiene.

Chapter 4

How to make your own Face mask

It's difficult to keep your distance in a grocery store or pharmacy during a pandemic such as the Covid-19, so now the CDC says we should wear a homemade mask in public to slow the spread of the coronavirus — particularly in areas with high community transmission.

Officials don't want healthy people using medical masks because of fears they would buy them all (kind of like toilet paper) and not leave them for health care workers.

We have the answer: Make your own.

The masks don't need to be professional-grade to help fight against airborne transmitted diseases such as Influenza and COVID-19. According to recent studies, the virus can spread between people in proximity by coughing, sneezing or even speaking.

It is important to note that covering your face with a piece of cloth won't protect you. But, it could help you from spreading the virus if you're like some people who lack symptoms and don't know they have it.

Sewing your own mask is easy, says Jeannette Childers, She's among scores of volunteers across the country sewing masks. So far, she's made so many for the Americans.

What is FFP protection classes

Aerosols and fine particles are two of the most treacherous health risks in a working environment and are nearly invisible in our breathing air. Filtering facepieces offer protection in three classes against these dangers: FFP1, FFP2 and FFP3.

Many dust masks bear the code FFP. This stands for 'filtering facepiece'. It shows what and how many particles of suspended dust, mist or fibres are filtered.

It isn't always easy to figure out all the different pictograms, standards and quality marks. With the right help, you can find the necessary information on every package so you always make the best choice at the building supply store. Always follow the instructions in the manual for correct use.

The importance of Filtering Facepieces respiratory protection

Dangerous particles can cause cancer or may be radioactive; others harm the respiratory system. Contact throughout decades may cause development of serious conditions. In the best case, all workers are confronted with are upsetting smells. Filtering facepieces offer protection in three classes against aqueous oily aerosols, smoke, and fine particles during work. Their protective function conforms to EU norm EN 149. This kind of facepiece is also known as particle-filtering half mask or fine particle mask and they are divided into the protection classes FFP1, FFP2 and FFP3.

How does a respirator mask work?

Filtering facepieces protect from respirable dust, smoke, and aqueous fog (aerosols), however they offer no protection from vapor and gas. The classifying system consists of the three FFP classes, the abbreviation FFP stands for "filtering facepiece". A respirator mask covers mouth and nose and is constructed of various filter materials and the mask itself. Their use is mandatory in working environments exceeding the occupational exposure limit value (OEL). This is the maximal concentration of dust, smoke, and/or aerosols in our breathing air that won't result in harm to health. In case of transgression, respirator masks must be worn.

Against what do respirator masks protect?

Depending on the total leakage and filtering of particle sizes up to 0.6 µm, respirator masks ranging from FFP1 through FFP2 to FFP3 offer breathing protection for various concentrations of pollutants. The total leakage comes about based on the filter penetration and leakages in the mouth and nose area. Our uvex respirator masks aim to avoid these by adapting our masks to human anatomy. Thanks to innovative filter technology, the breathing resistance can be held minimal and breathing isn't exacerbated intercepted particles in the filter after multiple-time wearing.

FFP1

- protection from atoxic and non-fibrogenic kinds of dust
- inhaling may result in development of health conditions; can also irritate the respiratory system and cause unpleasant odors
- total leakage may amount to a maximum of 25 %

- this kind of mask may be applied under a fourfold OEL transgression at the most

Protection class FFP1 respirator masks are made for working environments in which neither poisonous nor fibrogenic kinds of dust and aerosols are to be expected. They filter at least 80 % of the particles measuring up to 0.6 µm and may be worn as long as the maximum workplace concentration transgression measures no more than the fourfold value. The building or food industry put FFP1 respirator masks to use in many cases.

FFP2

- protection from firm and fluid deleterious kinds of dust, smoke, and aerosols
- particles may be fibrogenic – which means they irritate the respiratory system in the short term and can result in reduction of elasticity of pulmonary tissue in the long run
- total leakage may amount to a maximum of 11%
- OEL transgression to the tenfold value

Protection class FFP2 respirator masks are made for working environments in which deleterious and mutagenic particles can be found in the breathing air. Respirator masks of this class must contain at least 94 % of the particles measuring up to 0.6 µm and may be used in environments transgressing the OEL up to a maximum of the tenfold concentration. The same goes for the TRK value (technical reference concentration). Protection class FFP2 respirator masks are often worn in the metal and mining industry. Workers in these industries are frequently in contact with aerosols, fog and smoke that result in conditions of the respiratory system such as lung cancer in the long term. On top, they harbor the massive risk of secondary diseases and active tuberculosis of the lung. Our uvex filter system with a layer of carbon protects wearers from unpleasant odors on top of the required breathing protection.

FFP3

- protection from poisonous and deleterious kinds of dust, smoke, and aerosols
- when working with oncogenic or radioactive substances or pathogens such as viruses, bacteria and fungal spores FFP3-class respirator masks are recommended
- total leakage may amount to a maximum of 5%
- OEL transgression to the thirtyfold value

Protection class FFP3 respirator masks offer maximum protection from breathing air pollution. The total leakage may amount to a maximum of 5% and they must filter 99% of all particles measuring up to 0.6 μm. This kind of mask also filters poisonous, oncogenic and radioactive particles. Protection class FFP3 masks are used in working environments transgressing the OEL by the thirtyfold industry-specific values. They are often used in the chemistry industry.

How to do Your homemade face mask?

The masks don't need to be professional-grade to help fight against FLU and COVID-19. According to recent studies, the virus can spread between people in proximity by coughing, sneezing or even speaking.

It is important to note that covering your face with a piece of cloth won't protect you. But, it could help you from spreading the virus if you're like some people who lack symptoms and don't know they have it.

Sewing your own mask is easy, says Jeannette Childers, who's 77 and lives in Mesa, Arizona. She's among scores of volunteers across the country sewing masks. So far, she's made 65.

What type of ties do you want?

There are three main ways we recommend tying the mask to your face, and you'll want to plan it out before starting.

Ties that go around your ears. These are loose ties that you tie together behind your ears each time you put the mask on. This is simplest to make and requires the least work up front, but you'll need to tie the mask each time you wear it. You can't simply slip it on.

Ear loops. Elastic may be better than fabric for this style, since you'll need the ties to be short and tight enough to stay securely wrapped around your ears, but not so short and tight that they pop off.

Ties that go around the back of your head. You'll want the ties to be long enough to go around the back of your head horizontally, but short enough that the fit won't be too loose.

What you'll need

- Fabric. You'll need enough to make two 12″-by-6″ rectangles (the size of the template below.) Use a tightly woven fabric. Cotton-blend t-shirts and pillowcases are good bets.
- Scissors to cut the fabric.
- Something to tie the mask on. This could be elastic, strips of fabric, or something such as shoelaces.
- Needle and thread. If you don't have any, there are still options.

Homemade face mask type 1

Materials

Front: 100% unused cotton fabric–no metallic fabrics Back:100% unused cotton or cotton flannel Attachment:1/8", 1/4",or 3/8" flat elastic (white is preferred, black is OK) OR Four 15" x 1/4" inch bias-tape style ties (no raw edges, white/light preferred, black/dark OK

(Note:The instructions list three sizes: Small, Medium, and Large. We would recommend making Small-and Medium-sized masks primarily.

If possible, making a few Large masks would be helpful as well. See instructions for cutting sizes below.)

1)Cut two rectangles of fabric, one for the inside, one for the outside.

a. Small: 7.5 x 5inches
b. Medium: 9 x 6 inches
c. c.Large: 10 x 7 inches

2) Cut elastic or ties. All ties can be ¼" x 15". You will need 4 for each mask (one for each corner). Elastic should be cut as follows. You will need 2 pieces for each mask.

a. Small: 6.5 inches
b. Medium: 7 inches
C. Large: 7.5 inches

3) Put right sides of cotton mask fabric together.

4) Starting at the center of bottom (long) edge, sew to the first corner, stop. Sew a piece of elastic or a fabric tie into the corner. A few stitches forward and back will hold this.

5) Sew to the next corner, stop, and bring the other end of that same elastic to the corner and sew a few stitches forward and back.If you are using fabric ties, add a new tie.

6) Now sew across that top of the mask to the next corner. Again put a 7" length of elastic in the corner (or a new tie)

7) Sew to the next corner and sew in the other end of the same elastic (or a new tie).

8) Sew across the bottom leaving about 1.5" to 2" open. Stop, cut the thread.

9) Turn mask right-sideout.

10) Pin 3 tucks on each side of the mask. Make sure the tucks are in the same direction. There must be 3 tucks to ensure a tight fit on the face.

11) Sew around the edge of the mask twice.

12)When you have finished your masks, please use a Sharpie marker to mark a 1" tall S, M, or L on the lower left corner of the insideof each mask to indicate the size. This will help providers select the correct size. If you do not have a Sharpie, please somehow designate size for the masks before you drop them off.

Homemade face mask type 2

Supplies and tools

This is a relatively simple project so it doesn't require a lot of materials and tools to be completed. You need:

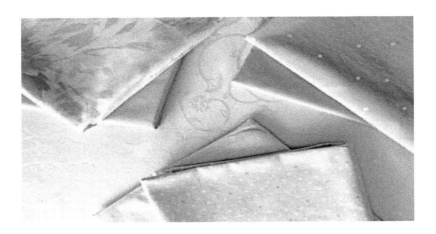

Face mask materials

- main fabric – about 13"x 7", cotton – all white or medical themed (tightly woven cotton, such as quilting cotton or cotton used in quality bed sheets)
- lining fabric about 13" x 6", cotton (tightly woven)
- filter (optional)
- 1/16" round elastic (preferable, currently available option , 1/8" or 1/4" flat elastic
- scissors (or better yet rotary cutter and a cutting mat)
- iron and ironing board
- sewing clips or pins
- a sewing machine (I recommend this one this one for beginners as it gets the work done and is reasonably priced or needle and a thread if you are handsewing

INSTRUCTIONS:

1. View the pattern and cut the fabric

face mask pattern and supplies on the cutting mat, Its original dimensions are 8.5 x 11 inches, which is about the size of a letter, small enough for easy printing. If you are not sure whether the dimensions are right, there is a small test square – 1 inch x 1 inch (US) and 2cm x2cm (for those outside US) on it so go ahead and measure it.

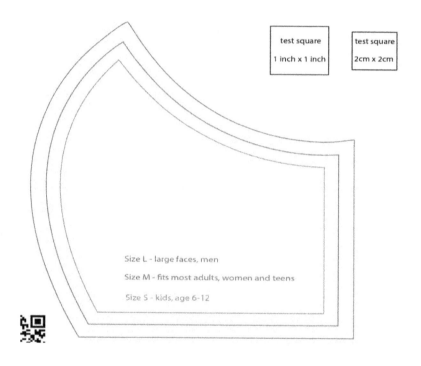

test square

1 inch x 1 inch

test square

2cm x 2cm

Size L - large faces, men

Size M - fits most adults, women and teens

Size S - kids, age 6-12

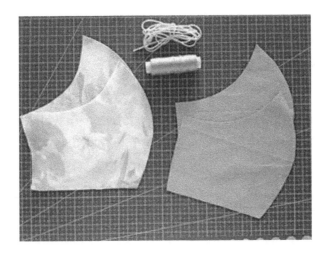

Download the pattern, print it out, and cut it accordingly. Before you put it onto your main fabric to cut it, fold the fabric in half so that the wrong sides are facing each other. Pin the pattern onto this folded fabric and cut the fabric just like the picture above.

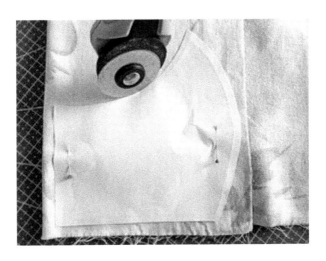

The seam allowance is 1/2 inch and is already included on all sides except for the ear side where you should add additional one inch seam allowance.

Repeat this step with the lining fabric as well. This time, however, do not add a seam allowance for the ear section.

TIPS: Several seamstresses asked us for fabric recommendations. Basically any thickly-woven cotton is fine and it is even better if you can add a filter medium

I saw someone wearing a stethoscope fabric mask and though that this is a great way to show appreciation to our front-liners. So, I found some suitable fabrics that can be purchased online. If you spot a great design, you can let your friends know

2. Sew the curve line of the face mask

Turn both pieces over and set them so that the right sides are on each other.

Sew along the curved line on both pieces.

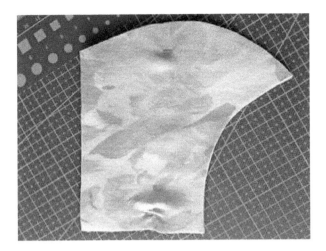

Then draw a line quarter-inch away from the original side line, on the inner layer. Do this for both side seams of the inner layer.

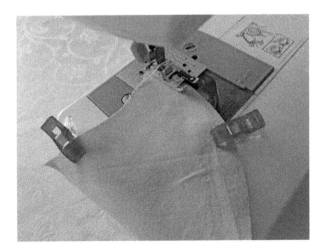

Next, you will need to clip the seam allowance on the curve part of the mask half an inch apart, both on the outer and the inner layer. Doing this allows the edge to stretch nicely instead of bulking up when you flip it inside out.

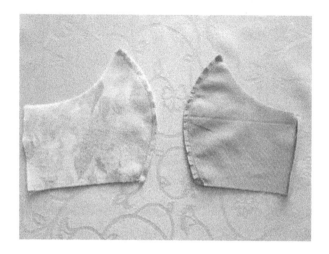

Now turn both pieces inside out and use the iron to press the seam allowances to different sides. If you want your mask to have a more professional look, topstitch near the seam line so that the seam allowances stay flat. Fold the side at the line you drew earlier and put the raw edge inside to hide it before topstitching it in place. Do this on each of the ear sides of the inner layer.

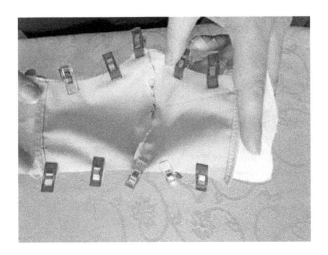

It's time to join the two layers together now. Put the inner layer on top of the outer, right sides facing each other so that the upper and lower edges align. Make a stitch at the bottom and top seam lines. If you did everything right up to this point, you will find that the edge of the outer layer is a about an inch away from the side seam line on the inner layer. If this isn't the case, retrace your steps and see where you made a mistake so that you can fix it.

Clip that curve on the seam allowance where the two layers meet and leave about half of an inch from the ends untouched. Flip the mask inside out again. Press the seams flat.

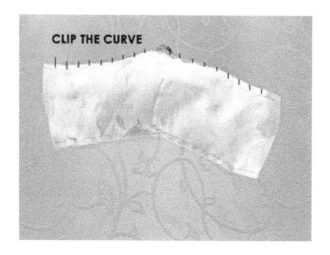

Fold the top and bottom raw edges of the outer layer twice and topstitch along the edge. Do this on the bottom seam line as well.

3.Add the elastic band and finalize your mask

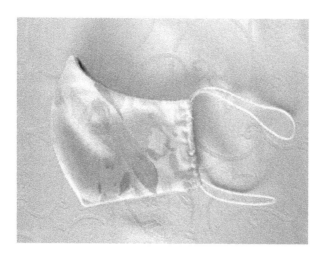

final face mask with elastic - ready to insert the filter

Now you will be making a channel for the elastic band. Fold the raw edge of the outer layer about a quarter of an inch away from the edge. Fold once again until that edge meets the edge of the inner layer.

Topstitch a vertical line across the part you just folded and you will be left with a vertical tube through which you can pull the elastic band.

– For 2 separate ear loops – you'll need 2 x 6"-8" of elastic for the adult sizes or 2 x 5 – 5 1/2" (kids)

– For one continuous piece that goes around the head – use 1 x 15-17" of elastic (again, depending on the size of the face)

TIP: Many makers report shortage of thin round elastic. You can use hair ties , ribbons or even make ties out of fabric.

4. Insert flexible nose wire (Optional)

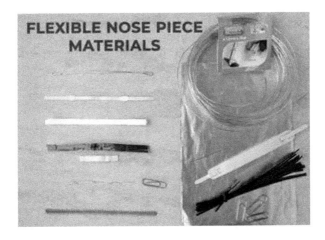

The mask will fit your face more closely if you add a flexible nose piece and mold it over your nose. I suggest using a 7″ long crafting wire or couple of twist ties, but as those are not always available, we get creative.

We've compiled our ideas and feedback from our readers and got to work. We tested which are the most suitable materials and what is the best length for the nose piece. Here's what we found – the most suitable materials for nose wire.

5. Insert filter (optional) and use the mask

You will also notice an opening between the outer and inner layers. This is where you can put the filter in. Change it regularly and keep your mask clean by washing it in the washing machine after each use.

What to use as a FILTER.

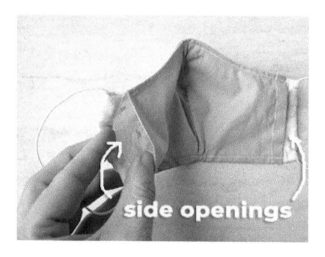

Note that these are not medically rated and their ability to protect is unknown:

As far as the filter goes you may use a piece of vacuum cleaner bag or HEPA filter without fiberglass, non woven fabric, or even an air-dried anti-bacterial wet wipe as filter. While those won't be able to stop the virus, they will be able to filter out more particles than fabrics alone. It probably all boils down to finding a balance between breath-ability and filtering. You'll have to make your own call here, and it would be smart to research whether and what filter to use.

Many readers asked why use vacuum dustbags as filter? According to this 2013 Cambridge university study which evaluated the capacity of several household materials to block bacterial and viral aerosols, vacuum cleaner bags were considered the most formidable household material with a rate of nearly 86 percent protection against the smallest particles they tested.

When placing the filter inside, make sure that it isn't crumbled up and that it reaches all the way to the upper edge. Once you put the mask on, make sure that it covers your nose well and that there are no gaps between your face and the mask.

Homemade face mask type 3

CDC recommends wearing cloth face coverings in public settings where other social distancing measures are difficult to maintain (e.g., grocery stores and pharmacies), especially in areas of significant community-based transmission.

CDC also advises the use of simple cloth face coverings to slow the spread of the virus and help people who may have the virus and do not know it from transmitting it to others. Cloth face coverings fashioned from household items or made at home from common materials at low cost can be used as an additional, voluntary public health measure.

Cloth face coverings should not be placed on young children under age 2, anyone who has trouble breathing, or is unconscious, incapacitated or otherwise unable to remove the mask without assistance.

The cloth face coverings recommended are not surgical masks or N-95 respirators. Those are critical supplies that must continue to be reserved for healthcare workers and other medical first responders, as recommended by current CDC guidance.

Sewn Cloth Face Covering

Supplies needed to create a cloth face covering are displayed. The supplies pictured include: one sewing machine, one twelve-inch ruler, one pencil, two six inch pieces of elastic string, two rectangle pieces of cotton cloth, 1 sewing needle, 1 bobby pin, 1 spool of thread, and 1 pair of scissors.

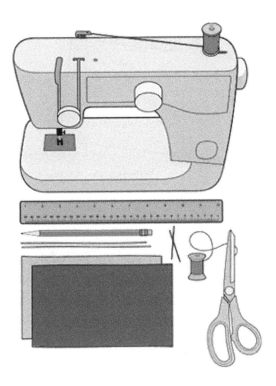

Materials

- Two 10"x6" rectangles of cotton fabric
- Two 6" pieces of elastic (or rubber bands, string, cloth strips, or hair ties)
- Needle and thread (or bobby pin)
- Scissors
- Sewing machine

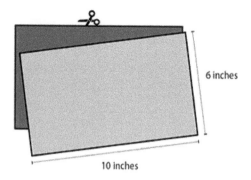

6 inches

10 inches

Tutorial

1. Cut out two 10-by-6-inch rectangles of cotton fabric. Use tightly woven cotton, such as quilting fabric or cotton sheets. T-shirt fabric will work in a pinch. Stack the two rectangles; you will sew the mask as if it was a single piece of fabric.

A close up of the two rectangular pieces of cloth needed to make a cloth face covering is shown. These pieces of cloth have been cut using a pair of scissors. Each piece of cloth measures ten inches in width and six inches in length.

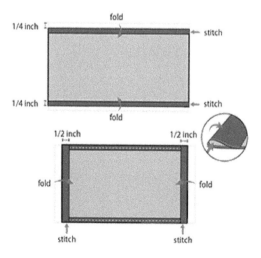

2. Fold over the long sides ¼ inch and hem. Then fold the double layer of fabric over ½ inch along the short sides and stitch down.

The top diagram shows the two rectangle cloth pieces stacked on top of each other, aligning on all sides. The rectangle, lying flat, is positioned so that the two ten inch sides are the top and the bottom of the rectangle, while the two six inch sides are the left and right side of the rectangle. The top diagram shows the two long edges of the cloth rectangle are folded over and stitched into place to create a one-fourth inch hem along the entire width of the top and bottom of the rectangle. The bottom diagram shows the two short edges of the cloth rectangle are folded over and stitched into place to create a one-half inch hem along the entire length of the right and left sides of the face covering.

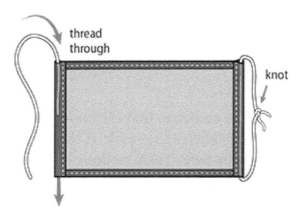

3. Run a 6-inch length of 1/8-inch wide elastic through the wider hem on each side of the mask. These will be the ear

loops. Use a large needle or a bobby pin to thread it through. Tie the ends tight.

Don't have elastic? Use hair ties or elastic head bands. If you only have string, you can make the ties longer and tie the mask behind your head.

Two six inch pieces of elastic or string are threaded through the open one-half inch hems created on the left and right side of the rectangle. Then, the two ends of the elastic or string are tied together into a knot.

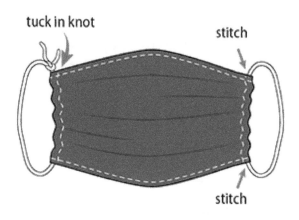

4. Gently pull on the elastic so that the knots are tucked inside the hem. Gather the sides of the mask on the elastic and adjust so the mask fits your face. Then securely stitch the elastic in place to keep it from slipping.

How to Wear an emergency Cloth Face Covering

Side view of an individual wearing a cloth face covering, which conceals their mouth and nose areas and has a string looped behind the visible ear to hold the covering in place. The top of the covering is positioned just below the eyes and the bottom extends down to cover the chin. The visible side of the covering extends to cover approximately half of the individual's cheek.

Cloth face coverings should :-

- fit snugly but comfortably against the side of the face
- be secured with ties or ear loops
- include multiple layers of fabric
- allow for breathing without restriction
- be able to be laundered and machine dried without damage or change to shape

Homemade face mask type 4

Assembly Guide Preparation

Fabric

This mask has two layers—the inner layer touching the face and the outer layer. The two layers can be made of the same fabric or different fabrics. Use 100% cotton or a cotton blend for the best filtration and breathability.

It takes two pieces of fabric about 14.5 in. x 7.5 in. (36 cm. x 18 cm.) to make one adult mask .

There are three sizes: Large, Medium, and Small. Patterns are available at the end of these instructions.

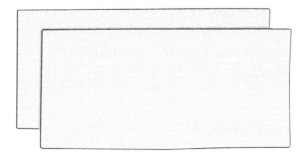

Ear Loop Material

Each mask needs two strips for ear loops. Ear loop material should be less than ½ inch (1.25 cm) wide. Some options are elastic, elastic cord, string, ribbon, bias tape, or even shoelaces.

If using elastic, each piece should be 12 inches (35.5 cm.) long. For other materials each piece should be 15 inches (38 cm) long.

Sewing Equipment

- Sewing machine
- Scissors or rotary cutter
- Thread
- Straight pins
- Safety pins

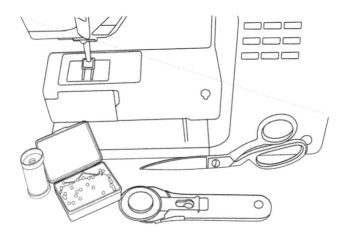

Work Area

Before you start sewing, ensure you are symptom free. Wash and sanitize your hands and your work area thoroughly with a disinfectant (it must indicate that it kills viruses) per the instructions on the label. Ensure there are no potential contaminants (e.g., pet hair, food, etc.) in the work area.

Assembly Guide Sewing Instructions

Step 1–Cut out the two main mask pieces.

- Fold the fabric in half. On the folded edge of the fabric, place the pattern edge marked "place on fold" .
- Pin the pattern on the fold of the fabric and cut it out.
- Repeat step 1 to cut the second piece.

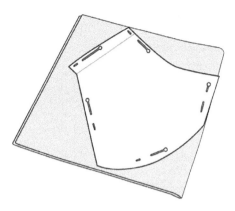

Step 2—Make the chin part of the mask.

- Open one of the cutout mask pieces. Fold it in half on the fold line, with the right sides inside.
- Sew along the chin seam, stitching 1/4 in (0.7 cm) from the edge .
- If desired, press the seam to the side to help it lay flat.
- Fold and sew the second mask piece in the same way.

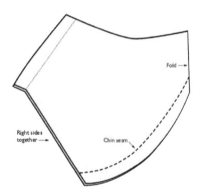

Step 3—Join the inner and outer layers together.

- Lay the two mask pieces on top of each other, with right sides of the fabric together .

- Sew the two layers together across the top of the mask, using a ¼ in (0.7 cm) seam.
- Sew the two layers together across the bottom of the mask.

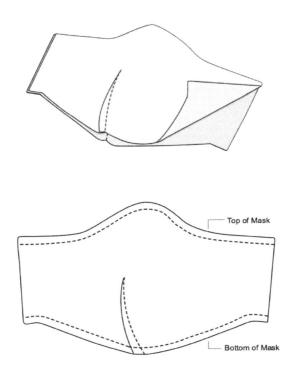

Step 4–Turn the mask right-side out.

- Press with an iron.

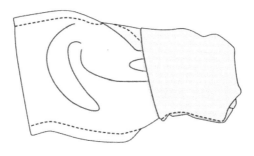

Step 5–Topstitch along the top and bottom edges.

- Keep your stitching close to the edges.
- Do not stich across the sides of the mask.

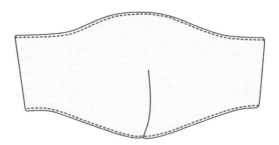

Step 6–Make the casing (a hollow channel) for the ear loop to go through.

On each side:

- Fold the raw side edges toward the inside of the mask about ¼ in (0.7 cm) (See Figure 10).
- Then fold over again, about 5/8 in (1.5 cm).
- Pin in place and stitch.

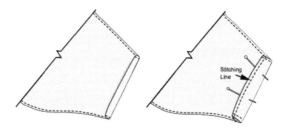

Step 7–Thread the ear loop through the casing along the sides of the mask.

- Use a large-eye plastic needle or attach the end of the elastic to a small safety pin. Push the elastic through the casing on both sides of the mask.

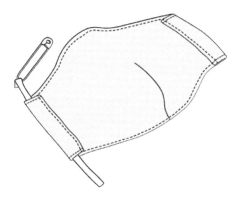

Step 8—Make loops the right size.

- Tie the loop ends loosely. The wearer can adjust the length by tying a knot.

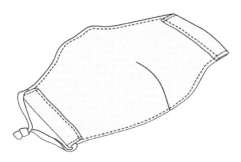

Large Face Mask

Sew with 1/4 in (6 mm) seam allowance.

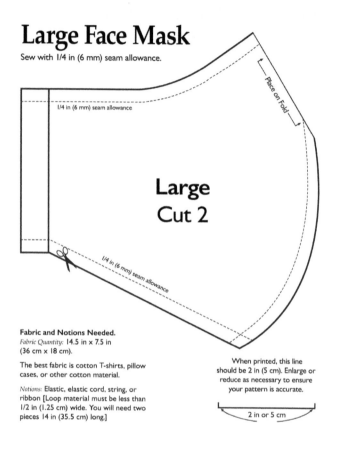

1/4 in (6 mm) seam allowance

Place on Fold

**Large
Cut 2**

1/4 in (6 mm) seam allowance

Fabric and Notions Needed.
Fabric Quantity: 14.5 in x 7.5 in
(36 cm x 18 cm).

The best fabric is cotton T-shirts, pillow cases, or other cotton material.

Notions: Elastic, elastic cord, string, or ribbon [Loop material must be less than 1/2 in (1.25 cm) wide. You will need two pieces 14 in (35.5 cm) long.]

When printed, this line should be 2 in (5 cm). Enlarge or reduce as necessary to ensure your pattern is accurate.

2 in or 5 cm

Medium Face Mask

Sew with 1/4 in (6 mm) seam allowance

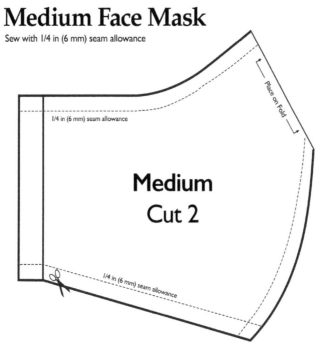

1/4 in (6 mm) seam allowance

Place on Fold

Medium

Cut 2

1/4 in (6 mm) seam allowance

Fabric and Notions Needed.

Fabric Quantity: 14.5 in x 7.5 in (36 cm x 18 cm).

The best fabric is cotton T-shirts, pillow cases, or other cotton material.

Notions: Elastic, elastic cord, string, or ribbon [Loop material must be less than 1/2 in (1.25 cm) wide. You will need two pieces 14 in (35.5 cm) long.]

When printed, this line should be 2 in (5 cm). Enlarge or reduce as necessary to ensure your pattern is accurate.

2 in or 5 cm

Small Face Mask

Sew with 1/4 in (6 mm) seam allowance

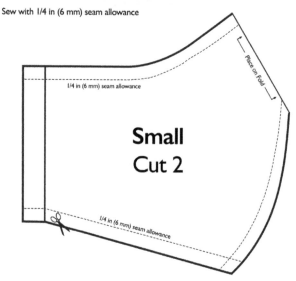

Fabric and Notions Needed.

Fabric Quantity: 14.5 in x 7.5 in (36 cm x 18 cm).

The best fabric is cotton T-shirts, pillow cases, or other cotton material.

Notions: Elastic, elastic cord, string, or ribbon [Loop material must be less than 1/2 in (1.25 cm) wide. You will need two pieces 14 in (35.5 cm) long.]

When printed, this line should be 2 in (5 cm). Enlarge or reduce as necessary to ensure your pattern is accurate.

2 in or 5 cm

Homemade face mask type 5

MATERIALS:

You will need:

- pieces of 100% cotton fabric 7" x 9"
- 2.2 pieces of 100% cotton fabric 1 ½" x 6"
- 3.2 pieces of 100% cotton fabric 1 ½" x 40"
- 4.Ruler
- 5.Pins
- 6.Scissors
- 7.Sewing machine & thread

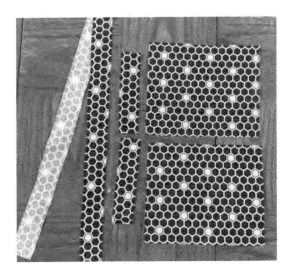

Masks should be constructed from tightly woven, high thread count cotton fabrics. The fabric should not have any stretch, and should not be knit (i.e. t-shirt material).

Recommended fabrics include: Poplin, Shirting, Sateen, and Percale in 100% cotton. A possible source of fabric is high thread count sheets and pillow cases.

Wondering if your fabric will work? A simple way to check is to fold it into two layers. You shouldn't be able to see through the fabric, but you should still be able to breathe if you hold it over your mouth.

Before you start, fabrics should be washed and dried on Hot in order to pre-shrink them.

INSTRUCTIONS:

1.Lay main mask pieces wrong sides together. Sew around edges at 1/4" to secure

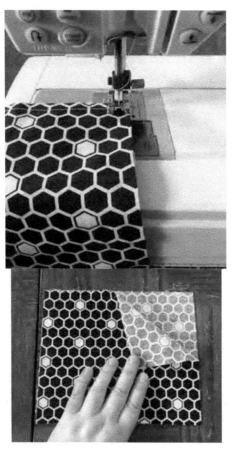

2.To create pleats: place pins along 7" edges as illustrated

3.Bring first needle to second to create pleat. Repeat with third & forth, fifth & sixth

4.Sew along previous stitching to secure pleats

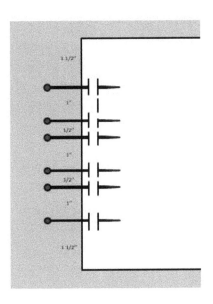

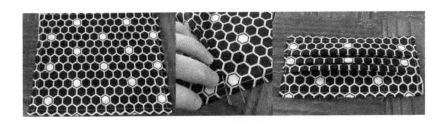

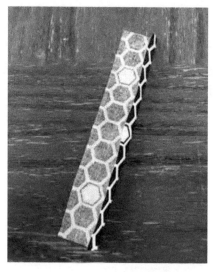

5. Press up 1/4" on both 1 ½" x 6" binding pieces

6. Lay unfolded side along pleated edge of mask, stitch at

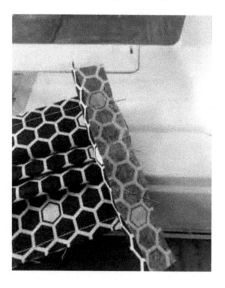

7. Fold binding around seam allowance & pin on opposite side, encasing raw edge. Topstitch in place.

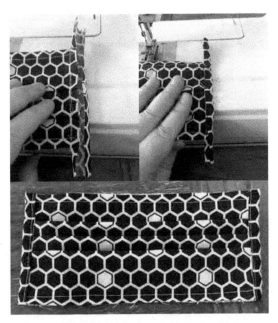

8.Repeat for opposite side. Trim binding to match mask

9.On both 1 ½" x 40" strap pieces, fold & press long edges to center

10.Fold the mask in half along the long edge & mark the center with a pin. Do the same with the strap

11.Matching centers, pin the strap in place. Stitch to mask body at 1/4" 12.Wrap strap around seam allowance as on binding & pin

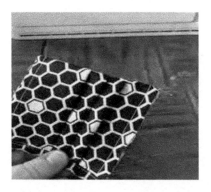

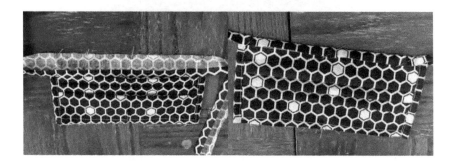

13. Unfold strap ends. Fold in 1/4", then re-fold pressed creases. Pin to secure

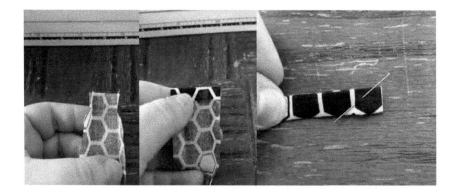

14. Top stitch along entire strap, including mask. To finish, stitch across strap ends to secure, and press pleats flat

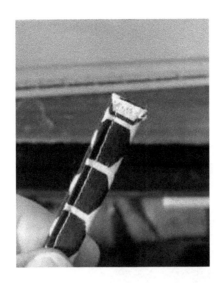

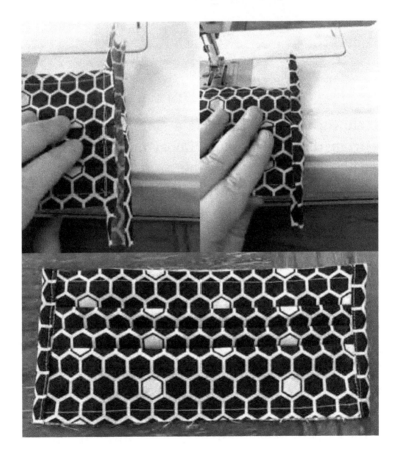

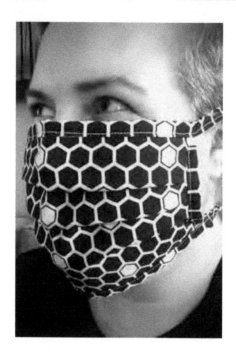

Three ways to upgrade the mask

We've shown you how to make a simple mask, based off of advice from the Pennsylvania Department of Health. But if you have a little more skill, here are three ways you can upgrade the mask:

Flip the mask inside-out instead of leaving the raw edges. Having the frayed edges inside could help keep the mask together and not degrade while being washed. It also looks nicer. To do this, first sew the ties to one layer, then layer the second layer on top of it. Then sew the two fabric layers together, leaving an inch or two of space instead of completing a full rectangle. Flip the mask inside-out through that rectangle, then sew around the outer edge again.

Fold horizontal pleats. This allows the mask to better fit the curvature of your face, similar to how surgical masks work.

The New York Times has a guide to making a mask with pleats and that you flip inside-out.

Use a third layer. Experts recommend having two layers of material, but some designs use a third, disposable layer to help filter air even further. Those can include materials such as Swiffer disposable dusting pads, coffee filters, paper towels, or something similar, said Suzanne Willard, associate dean of global health at Rutgers School of Nursing, who herself makes masks with disposable liners.

Some things to remember about your homemade mask

Disinfect the mask between every use. The easiest way is to wash it with the rest of your laundry, in hot water and with soap or detergent, and then run it through the dryer. You may want to make more than one mask, depending how often you go outside.

Take the mask off carefully. Wash your hands before taking the mask off and assume the virus is collected on the front of the mask. Don't touch the front directly, and instead take the mask off by the ties. Remember not to touch your face. Wash your hands after unmasking.

Masks don't provide perfect protection. Wearing a mask does not give you more freedom to come in contact with others or otherwise engage in risky behaviors. Continue to stay home as much as you can and maintain physical distance from others when you do go outside.

The mask should fit snugly around your nose and mouth. For an even better fit, you can sew a bendable piece of metal, such as a paperclip, to the top edge of the mask. That helps create a custom fit around the nose.

Do not touch the mask when in use, which risks transmitting the virus to your face.

Conclusion

Airborne diseases such as flu and COVID19 is spread from person-to-person in droplets of moisture, mucus and saliva from people with infections. Coughing, sneezing, and even normal breathing put these virus particles into the air. One sneeze can put out thousands of droplets.

People standing less than 6 feet away may become covered with these virus particles while they are still in the air. After the droplets fall, the virus particles can remain active for up to nine days.

Infection occurs when someone breathes in airborne droplets, or when they touch their mouth, nose or eyes with hands covered in virus particles that have fallen out of the air onto counters, hand rails, floors or other surfaces.

Wearing a face mask stops people from becoming infected in two ways:

1) By blocking most airborne droplets filled with virus from being inhaled

2) By stopping the wearer from touching their own mouths and noses.

Studies have shown that medical professional using surgical face masks correctly get 80% fewer infections than those who don't.

So why the mixed messages?

First, because the protection only comes when the masks are used properly. They must be put on clean, taken off carefully, and paired with rigorous hand washing, and the discipline not to touch the face.

Second, because gaps around the masks and between fibers, even in commercial surgical masks, are too large to block all viruses. Sneeze and cough droplets are usually between 7 and 100 microns. Surgical masks and some cloth masks will block 7 micron particles. The COVID19 virus particles are 0.06 to 0.14 microns.

So why should you make your own face masks?

1) In the event you become sick, having a supply of masks at home will give some level of protection to friends and family while you seek medical advice. It will certainly be better than no mask at all (see research notes).

2) By making your own, and hopefully for family and friends, you will be decreasing demand on limited supplies of industrially manufactured, disposables, which are desperately needed by hospitals and nursing homes.

3) These comfortable, curved shaped masks rest closer to the face, with fewer gaps, than rectangular surgical masks.

4) Our homemade designs are washable, making them environmentally friendly.

HOMEMADE HAND SANITIZER

By
Johnson Pfizer

Table of contents

Introduction

When it comes to preventing the spread of pandemic infectious diseases like COVID-19, nothing beats good old-fashioned handwashing.

But if water and soap aren't available, your next best option, according to the Centers for Disease Control and Prevention (CDC)Trusted Source, is to use an alcohol-based hand sanitizer that contains at least 60 percent alcohol.

Unless you have a stockpile of store-bought hand sanitizer, you'll likely have a hard time finding any at a store or online right now. Due to the rapid spread of the novel coronavirus, most retailers can't keep up with the demand for hand sanitizer, so the best option is for us to make our own homemade hand sanitizer. And that is what we are going to show you in this ebook. Sit back and enjoy as you learn one the most important prevention skill right now.

The good news? All it takes is three ingredients to make your own hand sanitizer at home. Read on to find out how.

Some commercial hand sanitizer contains ingredients as scary as the germs they protect you from, so why not make your own hand sanitizer from ingredients you select? This is an excellent project for kids as well as adults since the project can be expanded to include a discussion about hygiene and disinfection. You'll save money, protect yourself from germs, and can customize the scent of the hand sanitizer so it doesn't smell medicinal.

First off, it's important to note that hand sanitizer isn't the first strategy to prevent infection. Frequent and thorough hand washing with soap (for at least 20 seconds) is hands down the best method for reducing hand germs and curbing disease transmission, according to the Centers for Disease Control and Prevention (CDC). When soap and water aren't available, though, hand sanitizers can be used as an alternative.

The alcohol in hand sanitizers lends those products their microbe-busting power, and the CDC recommends that sanitizers contain 60% to 95% alcohol in order to eradicate germs. Sanitizers work best on clean hands and may be less effective when hands are greasy or visibly dirty.

Homemade hand sanitizers can also curb microbe exposure — but only as long as they have the correct ratio of alcohol to other ingredients.

"We know it works — just make sure it has enough alcohol in it.

You will surely be happy to buy this ebook on how to make you own sanitizer from home.

Chapter 1

What you need to know about homemade sanitizer

You probably haven't considered making your own hand sanitizer. Stores sell it for cheap, in a variety of scents and styles, and it's basically as good as it can be. But if you've been to a pharmacy in the midst of a viral outbreak like the one currently gripping the nations across the world, you've likely noticed that shelves empty as anxiety levels rise.

Right now in New York City, for example, it's not easy to get any disinfectant product (wipes, spray, etc.), and the fish bowls full of hand sanitizer bottles you would normally find at the checkout counter aren't even there anymore.

So, if that old bottle of hand sanitizer you've been carrying around is half-empty, don't panic. You can make your own sanitizing gel with supplies you can find at a drugstore or may already have at home.

There are two main formulas out there: one, recommended by the World Health Organization, is closer to liquid than gel and is harder on your hands, while the other will be gentler on your skin and closely resembles the feel of store-bought hand sanitizer. Which one you make depends on your personal preference.

But before you start, it's crucial that you understand simply rubbing your paws with hand sanitizer is not a substitute for good hand washing. Alcohol-based disinfectants used in the right amount (3 milliliters) and rubbed long enough (25 to 30 seconds) are fine in a pinch, because you're not always near a sink. But soap, water, and a good scrub is the absolute best way to protect yourself against contagious diseases. Got it? Good. Let's do this.

Hand Hygiene

Handwashing is one of the best ways to protect yourself and your family from getting sick. Learn when and how you should wash your hands to stay healthy.

How Germs Spread

Washing hands can keep you healthy and prevent the spread of respiratory and diarrheal infections from one person to the next. Germs can spread from other people or surfaces when you:

- Touch your eyes, nose, and mouth with unwashed hands
- Prepare or eat food and drinks with unwashed hands
- Touch a contaminated surface or objects
- Blow your nose, cough, or sneeze into hands and then touch other people's hands or common objects

Key Times to Wash Hands

You can help yourself and your loved ones stay healthy by washing your hands often, especially during these key times when you are likely to get and spread germs:

- Before, during, and after preparing food
- Before eating food
- Before and after caring for someone at home who is sick with vomiting or diarrhea
- Before and after treating a cut or wound
- After using the toilet
- After changing diapers or cleaning up a child who has used the toilet
- After blowing your nose, coughing, or sneezing
- After touching an animal, animal feed, or animal waste
- After handling pet food or pet treats
- After touching garbage

Follow Five Steps to Wash Your Hands the Right Way

Washing your hands is easy, and it's one of the most effective ways to prevent the spread of germs. Clean hands can stop germs from spreading from one person to another and throughout an entire community—from your home and workplace to childcare facilities and hospitals.

Follow these five steps every time.

- Wet your hands with clean, running water (warm or cold), turn off the tap, and apply soap.
- Lather your hands by rubbing them together with the soap. Lather the backs of your hands, between your fingers, and under your nails.
- Scrub your hands for at least 20 seconds. Need a timer? Hum the "Happy Birthday" song from beginning to end twice.
- Rinse your hands well under clean, running water.
- Dry your hands using a clean towel or air dry them.

Why should you take care of your hand?

Keeping hands clean is one of the most important steps we can take to avoid getting sick and spreading germs to others. Many diseases and conditions are spread by not washing hands with soap and clean, running water.

How germs get onto hands and make people sick

Feces (poop) from people or animals is an important source of germs like Salmonella, E. coli O157, and norovirus that cause diarrhea, and it can spread some respiratory infections like adenovirus and hand-foot-mouth disease. These kinds of germs can get onto hands after people use the toilet or change a diaper, but also in less obvious ways, like after handling raw meats that have invisible amounts of animal poop on them. A single gram of human feces—which is about the weight of a paper clip—can contain one trillion germs [1]. Germs can also get onto hands if people touch any object that has germs on it because someone coughed or sneezed on it or was touched by some other contaminated object. When these germs get onto hands and are not washed off, they can be passed from person to person and make people sick.

Washing hands prevents illnesses and spread of infections to others

Handwashing with soap removes germs from hands. This helps prevent infections because:

People frequently touch their eyes, nose, and mouth without even realizing it. Germs can get into the body through the eyes, nose and mouth and make us sick.

Germs from unwashed hands can get into foods and drinks while people prepare or consume them. Germs can multiply in some types of foods or drinks, under certain conditions, and make people sick.

Germs from unwashed hands can be transferred to other objects, like handrails, table tops, or toys, and then transferred to another person's hands.

Removing germs through handwashing therefore helps prevent diarrhea and respiratory infections and may even help prevent skin and eye infections.

Teaching people about handwashing helps them and their communities stay healthy. Handwashing education in the community:

- Reduces the number of people who get sick with diarrhea by 23-40% 2, 3, 6
- Reduces diarrheal illness in people with weakened immune systems by 58% 4
- Reduces respiratory illnesses, like colds, in the general population by 16-21% 3, 5

- Reduces absenteeism due to gastrointestinal illness in schoolchildren by 29-57% 7

Not washing hands harms children around the world

About 1.8 million children under the age of 5 die each year from diarrheal diseases and pneumonia, the top two killers of young children around the

world 8.

- Handwashing with soap could protect about 1 out of every 3 young children who get sick with diarrhea 2, 3 and almost 1 out of 5 young children with respiratory infections like pneumonia 3, 5.
- Although people around the world clean their hands with water, very few use soap to wash their hands. Washing hands with soap removes germs much more effectively 9.
- Handwashing education and access to soap in schools can help improve attendance 10, 11, 12.
- Good handwashing early in life may help improve child development in some settings 13.
- Estimated global rates of handwashing after using the toilet are only 19% 6.

Handwashing helps battle the rise in antibiotic resistance

Preventing sickness reduces the amount of antibiotics people use and the likelihood that antibiotic resistance will develop. Handwashing can prevent about 30% of diarrhea-related sicknesses and about 20% of respiratory infections (e.g., colds) 2, 5. Antibiotics often are prescribed unnecessarily for these health issues 14. Reducing the number of these infections by washing hands frequently helps prevent the overuse of antibiotics—the single most important factor leading to antibiotic resistance around the world. Handwashing can also prevent people from getting sick with germs that are already resistant to antibiotics and that can be difficult to treat.

Chapter 2

What is Hand sanitizer?

Throughout the day, people are exposed to thousands of types of germs. Illness like the cold and flu can be easily spread without the right precautions. When you come in contact with an item contaminated with germs and then touch your face, you may be vulnerable to illness. Fortunately, you can take steps to protect yourself simply by applying hand sanitizer.

Hand sanitizer is a product that is applied to the hands. Although their formulas vary, hand sanitizers typically contain active ingredients called antimicrobials. When applied to the skin, antimicrobials kill bacteria and in some cases, other types of germs. Using a hand sanitizer regularly can minimize the risk of illness and lower the likelihood of you spreading germs to your family, friends and coworkers. Unlike hand soap, hand sanitizer does not need to be rinsed after application, making it convenient to use on the go.

Some hand sanitizers leave behind a pleasing fragrance similar to hand lotion and hand soap. Manufacturers often offer their product in a number of different fragrances, giving you the ability to choose the option that is most pleasing to you. For those with sensitive skin or that do not want the added benefits of fragrance, there are also unscented hand sanitizer products

There are a number of features that you can consider when thinking of getting a hand sanitizer products. Liquid hand sanitizers can increase the risk of dry skin. If your hands are prone to dryness, you may want to opt for hand sanitizer wipes or look for liquids that contain moisturizing ingredients to counteract the drying actions of their formulas. Wipes are often a convenient choice for children, and individually wrapped ones are easy to carry in a diaper bag or purse when you are on the go. Some hand sanitizers contain anti-inflammatory ingredients like aloe vera and lavender to calm redness, itching and other signs of irritation.

Benefits and uses of hand sanitizer

This shouldn't come as much of a surprise. One of the foremost benefits of hand sanitizer is just that: It sanitizes. These products were designed to kill germs, and they get the job done. When used properly, hand sanitizers can eliminate 99.9% of the germs on your hands. The CDC recommends washing your hands any time you're around food (preparing it or eating it), animals, garbage, and more. When you find yourself in these situations, hand sanitizer is the perfect addition to (or occasional replacement for) washing your hands with soap and water.

Last time we checked, you can't take a sink on the go. In those situations where you need to wash your hands, there isn't always going to be soap and water available. You can slip a small bottle of hand sanitizer in your glove compartment, a purse, or even your pocket for situations where you might want to wash your hands but either can't find a sink or waiting for one is inconvenient (think long lines or far away restrooms). It's perfect for when you're grabbing a snack at a sporting event or have just left a public space, like the grocery store.

You know you need to keep your hands clean. As much as your hands serve you, they also put germs in contact with your mouth, eyes, nose, and many other parts of your body. We hope you're already washing your hands with soap and warm water multiple times a day, as that is the best way to clean them, but another worthy alternative is hand sanitizer. If you haven't already made this germ-fighter a staple on your shopping list, you may want to do so after learning about the benefits of hand sanitizer.

At the office, in the classroom, or in any space with lots of foot traffic, germs spread quickly. And even if you're not getting ready to eat or taking out the garbage, other people's germs can affect you (especially in close quarters). That's why having hand sanitizer available is ideal for group settings. Teachers, students, and office workers can kill germs periodically throughout the day without having to leave their classroom or desk, and gym-goers can use a squirt of hand sanitizer before hopping on the next workout machine.

Especially during flu season, minimizing your exposure to other people's germs is crucial for your health. When you take a moment to sanitize your hands a few times throughout the day, you reduce your chances of getting sick. Even a quick trip to a friend's house or the store can expose you to germs that could cause a cold, the flu, or other illnesses, so keeping your hands as clean as possible is important.

This might be one of the most surprising benefits of hand sanitizer, but it isn't too good to be true. Hand sanitizers that do not contain alcohol can actually improve the texture of the skin on your hands (note that hand sanitizers with alcohol won't have this effect). Some hand sanitizers contain emollients that soften your skin, giving you nicer-looking and smoother hands. You'll definitely notice a difference in how moisturized your skin feels and looks. Avoid hand sanitizers that contain alcohol, as they wash away the skin's natural oils and can cause the skin to crack, which in turns creates an entry point for bacteria.

How to use hand sanitizer in different settings

Hand sanitizer at health settings

Healthcare workers and patience may not be using the right amount of hand sanitizer or letting it dry on their hands long enough to achieve maximum protection against the spread of germs, a recent study suggests.

Researchers did lab tests to see how long different amounts of gel and foam versions of alcohol-based hand sanitizer took to dry on nine volunteers' hands. In the test of 0.75-milliliter, 1.5ml, 2.25ml and 3ml dollops, smaller amounts of sanitizer sometimes dried within the 20-30 second time frame recommended by the World Health Organization for optimal effectiveness, but none of the products dried that fast when the largest amounts were used.

"Some people with larger hands may need a bit more product, and this demonstrates that the amount being dispensed in many standard dispensers is not providing the ideal amount of product," said Elaine Larson, professor emerita at the Columbia University School of Nursing in New York City.

In the study, volunteers needed at least 2.25ml of sanitizer, and sometimes more, for optimal coverage on the front and back of hands.

Researchers also looked at how much hand sanitizer health workers and patience applied in real-world settings and compared how quickly workers thought it dried to actual drying times. Generally, workers thought sanitizer dried much faster than it really did.

"Staff have an unrealistic idea of the timing for hand hygiene," Larson, who wasn't involved in the study, said by email. "Alcohol is only active when it is wet so drying time is important."

To fight germs effectively, alcohol-based hand sanitizers should contain at least 60% alcohol, according to the U.S. Centers for Disease Control and Prevention. People should cover all surfaces of the hands, including spaces between fingers, and rub hands together for around 20 seconds, until hands feel dry, according to the CDC.

When hands are dirty or greasy, people should ideally wash hands with soap and water, and only use sanitizer when handwashing isn't an option.

Hand sanitizer in school setting

While there are some schools and correctional facilities that shy away from alcohol-based hand sanitizers, it isn't across the board. We have, in fact, seen significant results achieved with alcohol-based hand sanitizers in school settings. In one study conducted in schools published by the "American Journal of Infection Control," absenteeism caused by illness was 50.6 person lower in classrooms that used alcohol-based hand sanitizer regularly and implemented a hand hygiene education program vs. classrooms that did not.

Facilities make individual choices based on many factors, but experts like the U.S. Centers for Disease Control and Prevention recommend the use of alcohol-based hand sanitizers.

While there are non-alcohol formulations, our recommendations typically agree with the experts, especially since so many studies have proven their effectiveness.

Non-alcohol hand sanitizers are not effective at killing germs. We tested the "top" selling non-alcohol hand sanitizers and none of them met the 2-log germ kill U.S. Food and Drug Administration (FDA) requirement. If a facility cannot use alcohol-based hand sanitizers, they should not waste their resources on products that are not effective. They should instead invest in a liquid or foam soap that meets the FDA Monograph for antibacterial hand soaps.

Should Hand Sanitizer Be Placed In Schools, Prisons and Restrooms?

They are both necessary. A study by the American Society for Microbiology and the American Cleaning Institute (ACI), formerly the Soap and Detergent Association, shows that almost a quarter of men and women don't wash their hands in public restrooms. And 46 percent of people who wash their hands don't wash long enough to be effective, according to the most recent ACI Clean Hands Report Card. When that happens, germs are transferred from hands to other surfaces throughout the building.

We find that installing hand sanitizer dispensers at the restroom exit helps reduce the risk of germs leaving the restroom and improves the image of the facility. Because it is in the traffic flow, it is more likely to be used – even by those who choose to not wash.

Placement of dispensers is critical. The best place is inside the restroom, on the wall by the exit door, next to the door handle, 36- to 46 inches off the floor. That makes it conveniently accessible to encourage use. Hand sanitizers should never be placed near the soap dispensers at the sink, as placement there can be confusing to patrons.

It is not necessary to use both soap and hand sanitizer in the restroom if the soap is an antibacterial soap. If the soap is not antibacterial, then we do recommend using an alcohol-based hand sanitizer to provide better germ protection. Non-antibacterial soaps do not provide adequate germ-killing required to prevent the spread of disease-causing bacteria. Antibacterial soap and alcohol-based hand sanitizers provide the necessary 99.99 percent germ-kill required by the FDA respectively.

Type of Hand Sanitizer

Depending on the active ingredient used, hand sanitizers can be classified as one of two types: alcohol-based or alcohol-free. Alcohol-based products typically contain between 60 and 95 percent alcohol, usually in the form of ethanol, isopropanol, or n-propanol.[1,6] At those concentrations, alcohol immediately denatures proteins, effectively neutralizing certain types of microorganisms.[2,4,6] Alcohol-free products are generally based on disinfectants, such as benzalkonium chloride (BAC), or on antimicrobial agents, such as triclosan.[1,6,7] The activity of disinfectants and antimicrobial agents is both immediate and persistent.[1,3,8] Many hand sanitizers also contain emollients (e.g., glycerin) that soothe the skin, thickening agents, and fragrance.

Effectiveness of hand sanitizer

The effectiveness of hand sanitizer depends on multiple factors, including the manner in which the product is applied (e.g., quantity used, duration of exposure, frequency of use) and whether the specific infectious agents present on the person's hands are susceptible to the active ingredient in the product. In general, alcohol-based hand sanitizers, if rubbed thoroughly over finger and hand surfaces for a period of 30 seconds, followed by complete air-drying, can effectively reduce populations of bacteria, fungi, and some enveloped viruses (e.g., influenza A viruses). Similar effects have been reported for certain alcohol-free formulations, such as SAB (surfactant, allantoin, and BAC) hand sanitizer. Most hand sanitizers, however, are relatively ineffective against bacterial spores, nonenveloped viruses (e.g., norovirus), and encysted parasites (e.g., Giardia). They also do not fully cleanse or sanitize the skin when hands are noticeably soiled prior to application.

Despite the variability in effectiveness, hand sanitizers can help control the transmission of infectious diseases, especially in settings where compliance with hand washing is poor. For example, among children in elementary schools, the incorporation of either an alcohol-based or an alcohol-free hand sanitizer into classroom hand-hygiene programs has been associated with reductions in absenteeism related to infectious illness.10,11 Likewise, in the workplace, the use of alcohol-based hand sanitizer has been associated with reductions in illness episodes and sick days.12 In hospitals and health care clinics, increased access to alcohol-based hand sanitizer has been linked to overall improvements in hand hygiene.

An effective hand sanitizer has at least 60% alcohol content, but some products contain the alcohol substitute benzalkonium chloride, which isn't as good at killing germs.

As people continue to buy these less effective products, they could be putting themselves at risk without realizing it.

Alcohol-free sanitation products use benzalkonium chloride as an alcohol replacement, But the CDC warned consumers of this alcohol substitute because it's not as effective as alcohol itself at killing germs and may merely reduce the growth of new germs.

But these items are still selling out on online retailer like Amazon, or their prices are being hiked up, signalling consumer interest in the alcohol-free options As people continue to buy these less effective products, they could be putting themselves at risk without realizing it.

Although washing your hands with warm, soapy water for at least 20 seconds is the best way to protect yourself, sometimes hand sanitizer is needed in a pinch. According to the CDC website, an effective hand sanitizer has between 60% and 95% alcohol content .

On hand sanitizer labels, alcohol may be listed as "ethanol," "isopropyl alcohol," or "ethyl alcohol." As long as a product has the appropriate alcohol percentage, it's fine, regardless of other ingredients.

"If you drop below 60% [alcohol content], the effectiveness drops very dramatically , said " Miryam Wahrman , a biology professor at William Paterson University

But be wary of any hand sanitizers or sanitation products that say they contain an alternative disinfecting ingredient that's just as effective as alcohol, like coconut oil, because that's not the case.

Alcohol-free Hand sanitizer

Most alcohol-free products available today come in a water-based foam. The products contain the active ingredient Benzalkonium Chloride, a quaternary ammonium. Unlike alcohol-based products, alcohol-free hand sanitizers often contain less than a 0.1% concentration of Benzalkonium. They still provide the same level of protection. The rest of the solution is mainly water and will often be enhanced with skin conditioners such as vitamin E and green tea extract. It's non-flammable, and the low concentrations of Benzalkonium make it relatively non-toxic. However, these products are all recommended for external use only.

Alcohol-free hand sanitizers entered the market to address the concerns and complaints of gels. In many ways, they have succeeded. Typically, these solutions are much easier on the hands. They also pose much less of a threat in cases of accidental ingestion. Alcohol-free hand sanitizers are a low fire hazard and are non-damaging to surfaces. One other clear benefit is the extended protection that occurs. Alcohol-based product's ability to kill bacteria ends once the product has dried on the skin, but benzalkonium-based products continue to provide protection well after the solution has dried.

Active Ingredients in a Hand sanitizer

Depending on the active ingredient used, hand sanitizers can be classified as one of two types: alcohol-based or alcohol-free. Alcohol-based products typically contain between 60 and 95 percent alcohol, usually in the form of ethanol, isopropanol, or n-propanol. At those concentrations, alcohol immediately denatures proteins, effectively neutralizing certain types of microorganisms. Alcohol-free products are generally based on disinfectants, such as benzalkonium chloride (BAC), or on antimicrobial agents, such as triclosan. The activity of disinfectants and antimicrobial agents is both immediate and persistent. Many hand sanitizers also contain emollients (e.g., glycerin) that soothe the skin, thickening agents, and fragrance.

Chapter 3

What ingredients do you need?

Regular handwashing is one of the best ways to remove germs, avoid getting sick, and prevent the spread of germs to others. Whether you are at home, at work, traveling, or out in the community, find out how handwashing with soap and water can protect you and your family.

A number of infectious diseases can be spread from one person to another by contaminated hands. These diseases include gastrointestinal infections, such as Salmonella, and respiratory infections, such as influenza. Washing your hands properly can help prevent the spread of the germs (like bacteria and viruses) that cause these diseases.

Handwashing is one of the best ways to protect yourself and your family from getting sick. Learn when and how you should wash your hands to stay healthy.

How Germs Spread

Washing hands can keep you healthy and prevent the spread of respiratory and diarrheal infections from one person to the next. Germs can spread from other people or surfaces when you:

- Touch your eyes, nose, and mouth with unwashed hands
- Prepare or eat food and drinks with unwashed hands
- Touch a contaminated surface or objects
- Blow your nose, cough, or sneeze into hands and then touch other people's hands or common objects

When To Wash Your Hands

You should wash your hands thoroughly:

- after using the toilet or changing nappies

- before,during and after preparing food
- between handling raw and cooked or ready-to-eat food
- before eating
- after using a tissue or handkerchief
- before and after attending to sick children or other family members.
- after smoking
- after handling rubbish or working in the garden
- after handling animals

How To Wash Your Hands Properly

To wash hands properly:

- Wet your hands with clean, running water, turn off the tap.
- Apply soap and lather well for 20 seconds (or longer if the dirt is ingrained).
- Rub hands together rapidly across all surfaces of your hands and wrists.
- Don't forget the backs of your hands, your wrists, between your fingers and under your fingernails.
- If possible, remove rings and watches before you wash your hands, or ensure you move the rings to wash under them, as microorganisms can exist under them.
- Rinse well under running water and make sure all traces of soap are removed.
- Dry your hands using a clean towel or air dry them
- It is best to use paper towels (or single-use cloth towel).
- Dry under any rings, as they can be a source of future contamination if they remain moist.
- Hot air driers can be used.

An idea at home: give each family member their own towel and wash the towels often.

Importance of Hand sanitizer

If you think that hand washing is only for kids and health workers, think again. According to health experts, hand washing is the most effective way to prevent the spread of diseases and infections. They say that a number of infectious diseases such as pinworms, common colds, hepatitis A, meningitis, salmonella, and influenza can be prevented from spreading simply by washing your hands.

The importance of handwashing cannot be overemphasized as history tells us how sanitation and handwashing saved thousands of lives because an Austrian-Hungarian physician by the name of Ignaz Semmelweis insisted that student physicians in the hospital that he worked washed their hands before touching maternity patients.

Doctors' students had been working on corpses in an Anatomy class and then proceeded to perform their rounds in the maternity ward without washing their hands. This experiment proved successful when maternity deaths decreased fivefold. Yet it took 50 more years before hand washing would become the norm in the medical profession.

Why Should You Wash Your Hands?

1) Germs Make People Sick.

Germs gain access to the body as they are transferred from one person to another or from contact with contaminated surfaces. Once inside the body, the germs avoid the body's immune system and start producing toxins that make you sick.

Bacteria, viruses, and parasites are the most commonly known causes of food-borne diseases and food poisoning.

2) You Can't See Germs But They Are Everywhere.

Germs such as bacteria and viruses are microscopic and not visible to the naked eye. But just because you can't see them doesn't mean they aren't there. As a matter of fact, some bacteria reside on your skin and some live inside of you.

You may not be aware but germs commonly reside on everyday objects such as cellphones, office desks, toothbrushes, etc., and they can be transferred to your hands when you touch them.

3) Washing Your Hands Prevents The Spread Of Germs.

Properly washing your hands eliminates the dirt and germs that can be spread to others. People, especially kids, don't realize it but they frequently touch their eyes, nose, and mouth which give the germs access to the body and cause illnesses.

Washing your hands also helps prevent the spread of skin and eye infections. Simply washing your hands can help prevent the spread of bacteria such as MRSA (Methicillin-Resistant Staphylococcus Aureus), Clostridium difficile, E. coli and Salmonella.

4) Washing your hands keeps you healthy.

The major benefit of frequent hand washing is that it keeps you healthy. It also helps keep your environment clean which prevents germs from spreading to others. Properly washing and drying your hands will reduce your risk of getting sick with diarrhea and getting a respiratory illness.

5) Washing your hands saves you a hospital stay.

The healthier you are, the less likely you will have to spend on expensive medical treatment at a hospital or emergency care clinic. Washing your hands with soap and water is definitely an inexpensive means of preserving your health and the health of those around you.

Hand washing Versus Hand Sanitizer

As explained by Reynolds; So there you have it: Proper handwashing is the gold standard. Why is it better than hand sanitizer? "Data show that they're both effective at reducing germs, but handwashing actually kills germs, but it also physically removes much dirt, debris, and spores that could make you sick," Reynolds said. So in contrast to hand sanitizer, washing your hands does remove those pathogens like norovirus, Giardia, and C. difficile.

"Again, it's not the soap alone that kills the germs but the friction of lathering and washing away the organisms that makes handwashing more effective," Reynolds said. Washing with soap has been shown to be better than washing with water alone because it loosens the germs' ability to grip to the hands, making them easier to rinse away.

"Hand sanitizers have made their way into health care environments for a reason they're quick, easy, and effective if handwashing isn't an option at that moment," Reynolds said. And they are great to use on your way out of places where you'd pick up germs — like a subway, portable toilet, or petting zoo.

And of course, hand sanitizer is great if you're in a place where you don't have access to clean, running water, says Tetro. So keeping a little tube when you're traveling, especially in developing countries, is a great strategy to avoid disease. The only real downside of hand sanitizer is that it can really dry out your hands and lead to irritation if you use it frequently or your skin is sensitive, says Reynolds.

When and How to use Hand Sanitizer

When sanitizers first came out, there was little research showing what they did and didn't do, but that has changed. More research needs to be done, but scientists are learning more all the time.

The active ingredient in hand sanitizers is isopropyl alcohol (rubbing alcohol), a similar form of alcohol (ethanol or n-propanol), or a combination of them. Alcohols have long been known to kill microbes by dissolving their protective outer layer of proteins and disrupting their metabolism.

According to the CDC, research shows that hand sanitizer kills germs as effectively as washing your hands with soap and water—unless your hands are visibly dirty or greasy. They also don't remove potentially harmful chemicals.

Hand sanitizers also don't kill some common germs soap and water do eliminate, such as:

- Cryptosporidium
- Clostridium difficile
- Norovirus

While washing with soap and water is the recommended means to clean your hands, an alcohol-based sanitizer with 60-95% alcohol can be used when soap and water are not available. The use of alcohol-based hand sanitizers has increased in the health care field as well as the general public since 1995.

The use of hand sanitizers is convenient as you can transport small bottles into your pocket, purse, car or simply keep a small amount at your work station or desk and it takes you only about 15 seconds to clean your hands.

Making your own hand sanitizer is easy to do and only requires a few ingredients which we will later explain in this book.

Chapter 4

Homemade Hand sanitizer

Hands get dirty. In fact, your hands are the germiest part of your whole body. Washing your hands with soap and warm water is the best way to get your hands clean but unfortunately you can't always get to a sink. That's carrying an alcohol or Alcohol-Free Hand Sanitizer with you always is a very good idea.

Just think about all the thousands of things you touch every day, most of which have never been washed. Door handles, shopping carts, light switches, remote controls, computer keyboards, gas pump handles, escalator rails, vending machine buttons, toilet flush handles, elevator buttons, ATM and credit card keypads, money, your cell phone and, dirtiest of all, other people's hands. Yuck! So what are you doing to protect yourself?

Do you just whip out your bottle of hand sanitizer and squeeze out a blob? That should take care of all those germs, right? Wrong! Just step away from that antibacterial hand sanitizer you bought at the checkout lane and no one will get hurt.

Here's why you shouldn't be using commercial hand sanitizer:

Triclosan—any product with a label that says "antibacterial" likely contains triclosan. While triclosan does kill bacteria, it doesn't protect against fungi or viruses including the ones that put you in bed for a week. To make things even worse it also helps bacteria become resistant to antibiotics. Yep, it helps create superbugs. Oh yeah, it's also a neurotoxin, endocrine and hormone disrupter in case that sort of thing matters to you.

Parabens—conventional hand sanitizers are loaded with these chemicals. They are added to most personal care products that contain water to prevent microbe growth. Parabens have been linked to endocrine disruption, reproductive toxicity, immunotoxicity, neurotoxicity, skin irritation and even cancer. No thanks!

Synthetic Fragrance—if your hand sanitizer has a nice smell it's probably loaded with toxic chemicals. And because fragrance is considered proprietary, companies don't have to tell you what they actually are. The EWG has stated that "fragrance mixes have been associated with allergies, dermatitis, respiratory distress and potential effects on the reproductive system." Seriously??

Alcohol—if a hand sanitizer is alcohol based it must contain a minimum of 60% alcohol concentration and can contain much higher. Alcohol is very effective at killing bacteria, fungi and some viruses but the downside is that it's mostly...alcohol. Start noticing how often your kids have their fingers in their mouths or lick their fingers and you might reconsider. At school, most teachers require kids to use hand sanitizer before lunch and after every trip to the bathroom. That's a lot of opportunities to lick alcohol.So what's a farm girl to do? You guessed it—make your own homemade version without all the yucky stuff.

For our homemade version of hand sanitizer I turned to my trusty essential oils along with some other products you probably already have around your house. Here's what I use and why:

Essential Oils—the combination of EOs in this hand sanitizer protect against environmental and seasonal threats and promote healthy immune function.

Aloe Vera Gel—known for its healing properties, aloe vera is also antibacterial, anti-fungal and antiviral. It is a natural cleanser due to the presence of saponins.

Witch Hazel–astringent, antibacterial, antiviral, anti-inflammatory and antiseptic. Contains tannins which are very useful in protecting the skin against bacterial attacks.

Vitamin E–a fat-soluble antioxidant that is essential for the maintenance of healthy skin.

Water–used here to loosen the final product making it easier to pump out of the bottle.

Recipes for alcohol free hand sanitizer

Alcohol-Free Hand Sanitizer An awesome, bacteria-busting hand sanitizer that is alcohol, chemical and toxin-free. Love this!

Experts agree that washing your hands with soap and water is still the most effective way of killing germs and preventing the spread of germs to other people. Hand sanitizer should be used only when you don't have access to soap and a sink. But when we're out somewhere and there's no sink in sight, I'm glad my family has this alcohol, chemical and toxin-free hand sanitizer to help keep germs, bacteria and viruses at bay.

Alcohol-Free Hand Sanitizer

1/2 cup pure aloe vera gel

1/4 cup witch hazel

1/4 cup distilled water

20 drops melaleuca essential oil

15 drops lemon essential oil

15 drops white fir essential oil

1/2 tsp vitamin E (you can use 3 1000 IU softgels)

8 oz. glass pump bottle

Mix all ingredients in a small bowl. Put into glass pump bottle with a funnel, pushing mixture through with a spoon. Screw on pump top. Use as needed.

How do you make alcohol free hand sanitizer?

This recipe is free from alcohol and is super easy to make! You simply combine Aloe Vera, Alcohol-Free Witch Hazel and Essential Oils for the best great smelling hand sanitizer that exists! And You can also use the following ingredients for your foaming hand sanitizer with foaming container:

While most hand sanitizers contain either ethyl alcohol or isopropyl alcohol, alcohol-free hand sanitizers are also good. These usually contain antimicrobial compounds like benzalkonium chloride that provide a lasting protection against bacteria. But alcohol-free products aren't recommended by the CDC for fighting the novel coronavirus, because it isn't yet clear that it can be used successfully against SARS-CoV-2.

- 3 Tablespoons Aloe Vera
- 1 Tablespoon Alcohol-Free Unscented Witch Hazel
- 15 drops Young Living Thieves Essential Oil
- 5 drops Young Living Lemon Essential Oil

Recipes and how to make alcohol Homemade Hand Sanitizer

We actually have two recipes for you in this categories, The first is one you can make with stuff you likely already have in your cabinets and under the sink, so it's effective in emergency situations. The second recipe is more complex, but easy to make if you have the opportunity to do some shopping and planning ahead of time. Another note: A lot of these items are quickly going out of stock because of high demand. There's a higher chance of finding them at your local drug store, but your first priority is to stay indoors.

Potency Matters

You're going to need some alcohol. According to the Centers for Disease Control and Prevention, your sanitizer mix must be at least 60 percent alcohol to be effective. But it's better to get way above that aim for a minimum of 75 percent. A bottle of 99 percent isopropyl alcohol is the best thing to use. Your regular vodka and whiskey are too wimpy and won't cut it.

The Quick (Gel) Recipe

- Isopropyl alcohol
- Aloe vera gel
- Tea tree oil

Mix 3 parts isopropyl alcohol to 1 part aloe vera gel. Add a few drops of tea tree oil to give it a pleasant scent and to align your chakras.

The Better (Spray) Recipe

- Isopropyl alcohol
- Glycerol or glycerin
- Hydrogen peroxide
- Distilled water
- Spray bottle

The aloe mixture gets the job done, but aloe also leaves your skin annoyingly sticky. So, here's a recipe that's less sticky and more potent, based on the mix recommended by the WHO.

Mix 12 fluid ounces of alcohol with 2 teaspoons of glycerol. You can buy jugs of glycerol online, and it's an important ingredient because it keeps the alcohol from drying out your hands. If you can't find glycerol, proceed with the rest of the recipe anyway and just remember to moisturize your hands after applying the sanitizer.

How to Make Alcohol base Foaming Hand Sanitizer

Supplies:

- 3 Tablespoons Aloe Vera
- 1 Tablespoon Alcohol-Free Unscented Witch Hazel
- 15 drops Essential Oil
- 5 drops Lemon Essential Oil
- Foaming container

ingredients to make foaming hand sanitizer

Directions:

- If desired, print and attach a Foaming Hand Sanitizer Label on your container.
- In your foaming container, combined all of your ingredients.
- Shake gently until well combined.
- Use liberally as needed.

How to make gel alcohol base hand sanitizer

People who have tried to make their own gel-based hand sanitizers can tell you that classic gelling agents like gelatin or agar won't behave when mixed with the high concentrations of alcohol that you need to kill viruses and bacteria. These agents won't form a gel that's stable because polar alcohol groups interrupt the intermolecular bonds. Manufacturers get around this obstacle by using high-molecular-weight cross-linked polymers of acrylic acid. The covalent cross-links help make a viscous gel that's resistant to alcohol's disruption.

- isopropyl or rubbing alcohol (99 percent alcohol volume)
- aloe vera gel
- an essential oil, such as tea tree oil or lavender oil, or you can use lemon juice instead

The key to making an effective, germ-busting gel hand sanitizer is to stick to a 2:1 proportion of alcohol to aloe vera.

This keeps the alcohol content around 60 percent. This is the minimum amount needed to kill most germs, according to the CDC.

Appropriate quantity for Hand sanitizer recipe

What you'll need:

- 3/4 cup of isopropyl or rubbing alcohol (99 percent)
- 1/4 cup of aloe vera gel (to help keep your hands smooth and to counteract the harshness of alcohol)
- 10 drops of essential oil, such as lavender oil, or you can use lemon juice instead

Directions:

- Pour all ingredients into a bowl, ideally one with a pouring spout like a glass measuring container.
- Mix with a spoon and then beat with a whisk to turn the sanitizer into a gel.
- Pour the ingredients into an empty bottle for easy use, and label it "hand sanitizer."

Second steps to make your gel alcohol hand sanitizer formula:

- two parts isopropyl alcohol or ethanol (91 percent to 99 percent alcohol)
- one part aloe vera
- a few drops of clove, eucalyptus, peppermint, or other essential oil.

If you are making hand sanitizer at home, adhere to these tips:

1. Make the hand sanitizer in a clean space. Wipe down counter tops with a diluted bleach solution beforehand.
2. Wash your hands thoroughly before making the hand sanitizer.
3. To mix, use a clean spoon and whisk. Wash these items thoroughly before using them.

4. Make sure the alcohol used for the hand sanitizer is not diluted.
5. Mix all the ingredients thoroughly until they are well blended.
6. Do not touch the mixture with your hands until it is ready for use.

For a larger batch of hand sanitizer, the World Health Organization (WHO) has a formula for a hand sanitizer that uses:

- isopropyl alcohol or ethanol
- hydrogen peroxide
- glycerol
- sterile distilled or boiled cold water

Chapter 5

What you must know about Essential Oils

In addition to adding fragrance to your hand sanitizer, the essential oil you choose may also help protect you against germs. For example, thyme and clove oil have antimicrobial properties. If you are using antimicrobial oils, only use a drop or two, since these oils tend to be very powerful and might irritate your skin. Other oils, such as lavender or chamomile, may help soothe your skin. Tea tree oil is antimicrobial. A couple of drops may be added to the recipe, but it's important to note many people are sensitive to this oil, even when it's diluted.

- What they are
- How they work
- Types
- Benefits
- Uses
- Tips for choosing
- Safety

Essential oils are often used in aromatherapy, a form of alternative medicine that employs plant extracts to support health and well-being. However, some of the health claims associated with these oils are controversial.

This article explains all you need to know about essential oils and their health effects.

What are essential oils?

Essential oils are compounds extracted from plants.

The oils capture the plant's scent and flavor, or "essence."

Unique aromatic compounds give each essential oil its characteristic essence.

Essential oils are obtained through distillation (via steam and/or water) or mechanical methods, such as cold pressing.

Once the aromatic chemicals have been extracted, they are combined with a carrier oil to create a product that's ready for use.

The way the oils are made is important, as essential oils obtained through chemical processes are not considered true essential oils.

Summary

Essential oils are concentrated plant extracts that retain the natural smell and flavor, or "essence," of their source.

How Do Essential Oils Work?

Essential oils are most commonly used in the practice of aromatherapy, in which they are inhaled through various methods.

Essential oils are not meant to be swallowed.

The chemicals in essential oils can interact with your body in several ways.

When applied to your skin, some plant chemicals are absorbed.

It's thought that certain application methods can improve absorption, such as applying with heat or to different areas of the body. However, research in this area is lacking.

Inhaling the aromas from essential oils can stimulate areas of your limbic system, which is a part of your brain that plays a role in emotions, behaviors, sense of smell, and long-term memory.

Interestingly, the limbic system is heavily involved in forming memories. This can partly explain why familiar smells can trigger memories or emotions.

The limbic system also plays a role in controlling several unconscious physiological functions, such as breathing, heart rate, and blood pressure. As such, some people claim that essential oils can exert a physical effect on your body.

However, this has yet to be confirmed in studies.

How aromatherapy works

When you sniff an essential oil, your olfactory bulb fires off signals to the limbic system, the part of the brain that controls emotions—that's how scents affect your mood. Depending on the type of oil used, your blood pressure or heart rate may rise or fall, and your body may release certain hormones.

That said, you have to like an oil for it to have an optimal effect (why my husband wasn't rejuvenated by our grapefruited room). "Besides the physical reaction, a psychological one happens when you smell a scent," notes Adriane Fugh-Berman, MD, associate professor of pharmacology at Georgetown University Medical Center. She recalls dissecting cadavers in medical school, when professors dropped peppermint oil into the formaldehyde to mask the odor. "For years, the smell of peppermint reminded me of dead bodies!" she says. "I still have to buy nonpeppermint toothpaste."

Homemade Aromatherapy Disinfecting

With cold and flu season in high-gear, disinfecting the home may be in order. Disinfecting is different from cleaning because disinfectants kill bacteria so that it is unable to reproduce. Cleaning pretty much just moves it around the surface, but does not actually kill bacteria that may be present.

It is not uncommon for bleach to be used as a disinfectant. However, bleach can be very dangerous and I don't recommend it. In fact, one of the best reasons to make your own aromatherapy disinfectant spray is that the amount of chemicals found in most off- the-shelf cleaners is very high and can be dangerous.

Check out my recipe below to make your own homemade disinfectant spray — which includes two antibacterial essential oils. This recipe is easy and can leave your home fresh and bacteria-free.

Ingredients

Makes 16 ounces

- 2/3 cup high-proof of 60%n alcohol
- 1/2 cup white distilled vinegar
- 3/4 cup distilled water
- 30–40 drops tea tree essential oil
- 30–40 drops lemongrass essential oil
- 16-ounce spray bottle

Instructions

Make sure you use a clean spray bottle. It should not have any bleach or other product residue. A new bottle may be the best way to go, but regardless, just make sure it is clean. Pour the alcohol, vinegar and water into the bottle. alcohol is a great disinfectant. Just use the cheap stuff. While alcohol does not kill bacteria, it helps clean surfaces and it works to eliminate odors. Vinegar is next up and is a great option since it can help remove dirt and grime. Next, add the distilled water. Using distilled water is important because it is bacteria-free.

Now, let's add the essential oils. But what essential oils are good for disinfecting? Tea tree essential oil is my favorite since it is antibacterial. Tea tree oil has shown effective wound-healing properties due to its ability to fight infection that can be caused from bacteria. That is why it is a great option for your DIY disinfectant spray.

Lemongrass is known for its antibacterial qualities too. Studies have shown that it is effective at fighting methicillin-resistant Staphylococcus Aureus (MRSA) skin infections. This makes it a good choice for getting rid of bacteria that may be living on your kitchen countertops too.

Now that everything has been placed in the bottle, simple screw the cap on and shake well. It's important to clean the area first (you may even want to try making our second disinfectant below) so that you remove any visible waste particles. Next, rinse the area and dry it. Then apply the homemade disinfectant spray. Shake well before each use.

Homemade natural spray disinfectant

Some mothers are scared of using homemade Thieves Oil around children, especially young children under 3 years old. Unfortunately, many of the ingredients contained in it should not be used on small children. In fact, rosemary essential oil shouldn't really be used around kids until they are at least 5 years old. Some sources indicate that children under 18 months of age should not be exposed to clove or cinnamon essential oils while other places indicate to keep them away from your children until they are at least 3 years old (and then only recommend the oils be used in sprays and diffusers).

In the end, it all comes down to what your child's pediatrician recommends and what you feel comfortable exposing your child to. No pure essential oils of any kind should ever be put on your child's body or ingested. Adults should also be very careful about putting undiluted essential oils on their skin because they often burn, especially oils like clove and cinnamon.

So as an alternative for those who would like to disinfect the air but are concerned about their children in the house, here is an alternative recipe for a homemade natural spray disinfectant. This can be sprayed into the air of any room to combat germs, viruses, bacteria and on on. I have also included some variations of the recipe below which are more suitable for children under 3.

Avoid letting the droplets fall on polished wood surfaces, delicate materials or other objects and materials in the room which could be damaged by the water or other ingredients in this spray. Mixing in glass containers is best — but never metal.

This is an excellent resource for parents who want to use aromatherapy and essential oil blends for their children.

Ingredients

- 4 ounces water
- 2 ounces alcohol (or vodka)
- 20 drops thyme linalol
- 5 drops cinnamon
- 5 drops clove
- 10 drops tea tree
- 10 drops lemon

Directions

- Add all the essential oils to the alcohol and stir.
- Add the oil/alcohol mixture to the water and let sit for 24 hours.
- Pour mixture into a clean spray bottle and spray into the air as needed.

Recipe Variations For Children By Age:

Newborn — Use of the above oils is not recommended around children that young. Instead use 25 drops of Chamomile and

25 drops of Lavender. The solution may not be as effective but Chamomile is still an antibacterial and Lavender has antibacterial as well as disinfectant properties.

2-6 months old — Use 20 drops of Eucalyptus Radiata, 10 drops Chamomile, 10 drops Tea Tree Oil and 10 drops Lavender.

7 months to 1 year old — Use 20 drops Niaouli, 10 drops of Eucalyptus Radiata, 10 drops Tea Tree Oil and 10 drops Lavender.

2-3 years old — Use 10 drops Niaouli instead of clove and cinnamon oils. Ravensara can also be substituted or 5 drops of each used to replace clove and cinnamon. Niaouli contains extra anti-parasitic properties but both have antibacterial, disinfectant and antiviral properties.

3 years old and older — All oils okay for use as long as clove and cinnamon oils are only used in diffusers and room sprays.

Safety tips of hand sanitizer

Hand sanitizers can remove germs from your hands when you use these products as they are intended to be used. The question is, are they as safe and effective as people think they are?

Dangers Associated With Hand Sanitizer Use

For all the good that hand sanitizers can do, some medical professionals have expressed concerns about some of their ingredients, as well as how these products are used. It's important to understand the dangers they are trying to bring to light.

Risk For Alcohol Poisoning

Hand sanitizer poses a potential risk for alcohol poisoning, particularly for young children who are attracted to the fun scents and bright colors of many sanitizers. According to Dr.

Sanjay Gupta, a two-ounce bottle of hand sanitizer contains 62 percent ethyl alcohol, or the equivalent of four shots of vodka. At that concentration, even a small dose can be dangerous if ingested, leading to dizziness, slurred speech, headaches, and even brain damage or death in extreme cases.

Take These Steps To Reduce The Risk Of Alcohol Poisoning:

- Avoid using instant sanitizers whenever possible, and opt for regular hand washing instead.
- Use only a dime-sized amount of sanitizer; too much liquid may not evaporate quickly and could be licked off fingers or palms.
- Supervise children while using sanitizers to ensure they rub their hands until completely dry, and store the sanitizer out of their reach.

Concerns About Triclosan

Triclosan, an antibacterial agent used in some hand sanitizers, as well as other health and beauty products, also appears to pose some risk. According to a report published in the Washington Post, the FDA is taking another look at Triclosan because some scientific studies appear to raise questions about the chemical's potential to disrupt the human endocrine system.

Samuel S. Epstein, MD and Professor Emeritus at the University of Illinois School of Public Health, Chicago, points out other concerns about Triclosan:

- Triclosan persists in the environment and is one of the top 10 contaminents found in U.S. waterways.
- The chemical has been identified as a contaminent in umbilical chord samples, and it has also been identified in breast milk.

- Triclosan reacts with chlorinated water to produce chloroform gas.

Furthermore, M. Angela McGhee, Ph.D., Biology and Marine Sciences, warns that Triclosan is actually classed as a pesticide by the U.S. Enviromental Protection Agency. Dr. McGhee maintains that Triclosan is a chlorophenol, and chlorophenols possibly cause cancer in people. Despite these concerns, Triclosan still has FDA approval for use in hand sanitizer.

Potential For Antibiotic-Resistant Bacteria

According to Medical News Today, another concern about hand sanitizers is that over-reliance on these products could ultimately produce bacteria that are resistant to antibiotics. Medical News reports that a study of 161 long-term care facilities revealed that facilities which favored using hand sanitizer over traditional hand washing were more likely to experience outbreaks of norovirus.

Potential Danger For Kids

Kids lead with their senses. If something smells like candy, it must taste like it. And if it has glitter in it, it just might be pretty enough to eat. That's why hand sanitizer looks so delicious to them. But swallowing just two to three squirts of certain hand sanitizers can make them really sick – even to the point of alcohol poisoning. By taking some quick and easy precautions, you can help keep your kids safer.

Steps To Safety

Hand sanitizer is one of the most popular germ-fighting products out there, but it can be really dangerous if kids swallow it. Using the right amount of hand sanitizer the right way is important. Here's how:

Put a dime-sized amount on a child's dry hands and have them rub their hands together until they're completely dry.

Remind children to keep their hands out of their mouths after applying it.

Kids like to eat with their hands. Try to use soap and water to wash-up before meals and snacks so they don't get hand sanitizer in their mouths.

Supervise kids when they're using hand sanitizer, and teach older kids how to apply it properly on their own.

What To Do

Did you know most hand sanitizers contain 60% ethyl alcohol? That's stronger than the concentration in most hard liquors. To protect your kids in your home:

Keep hand sanitizer out of their reach and only allow them to use it when an adult is supervising them.

Avoid buying hand sanitizer that looks or smells fruity so your child will be less tempted to try a taste.

If you can, consider using sanitizing wipes, liquids or foams that are not alcohol-based.

During An Emergency

Symptoms Of Alcohol Poisoning

Can't think clearly

- Throwing up
- Can't stay awake
- Breathing slowly or irregularly
- Looking blue or pale
- Shivering

Call the Poison Help number right away if you think your child has swallowed hand sanitizer. Don't wait for symptoms to develop.

Call 911 if your child shows symptoms of alcohol poisoning.

Conclusion

The portable hand sanitizers do have a role during peak respiratory virus season because they make it much easier to clean your hands.

It's much more difficult when you sneeze to wash your hands than it is to use a hand sanitizer, especially when you are outdoors or in a car. The hand sanitizers are much more convenient, so they make it more likely that people will clean their hands, and that's better than not cleaning at all.

According to the Centers for Diseae Control (CDC), however, for hand sanitizer to be effective it must be used correctly. That means using the proper amount (read the label to see how much you should use), and rubbing it all over the surfaces of both hands until your hands are dry. Do not wipe your hands or wash them after applying.

It's important to make sure any hand sanitizer you do use contains at least 60 percent alcohol, unless you decided to go an alcohol-free hand sanitizer.

Studies have found that sanitizers with lower concentrations or non-alcohol-based hand sanitizers are not as effective at killing germs as those with 60 to 95 percent alcohol.

In particular, non-alcohol-based sanitizers may not work equally well on different types of germs and could cause some germs to develop resistance to the sanitizer.

There is no proof that alcohol-based hand sanitizers and other antimicrobial products are harmful.

They could theoretically lead to antibacterial resistance. That's the reason most often used to argue against using hand sanitizers. But that hasn't been proven. In the hospital, there hasn't been any evidence of resistance to alcohol-based hand sanitizers.

However, while there aren't any studies showing that hand sanitizers definitely pose a threat, there also isn't any evidence that they do a better job of protecting you from harmful bacteria than soap.

So while hand sanitizers have their place — in hospitals or when you can't get to a sink — washing with soap and warm water is almost always a better choice.

Lightning Source UK Ltd.
Milton Keynes UK
UKHW020653080221
378420UK00012B/873